Sound and Sense in Contemporary Theatre

Matthew Tomkinson

Sound and Sense in Contemporary Theatre

Mad Auralities

palgrave
macmillan

Matthew Tomkinson
Vancouver, BC, Canada

ISBN 978-3-031-78033-2 ISBN 978-3-031-78034-9 (eBook)
https://doi.org/10.1007/978-3-031-78034-9

This Palgrave Macmillan imprint is published by the registered company Springer Nature Switzerland AG
The registered company address is: Gewerbestrasse 11, 6330 Cham, Switzerland

For Elissa, who listened and laughed with me amid the breakdowns (there were some) and the breakthroughs (there were many).

Acknowledgements

I have been privileged to conduct research for this book project on the unceded territories of the xʷməθkʷəy̓əm (Musqueam), Sḵwx̱wú7mesh (Squamish), and səl̓ilwətaʔɬ (Tsleil-Waututh) Nations, where I am fortunate to live, dance, play music, and work as a settler scholar.

One would be hard-pressed to find an acknowledgements page that did not mention the writer's sanity and those who helped preserve it. Even more important to me are those who are able to hold space for the madness, whenever and however it shows up. I am lucky to have been surrounded by such gracious people throughout this process.

On that note, my first thanks go to my former supervisor, Dr. Kirsty Johnston, for her unflagging support and encouragement. I am extremely grateful for her mentorship, which has always been charitable, insightful, and rigorous. Endless thanks also go to Dr. Susan Bennett and Dr. Lisa Coulthard, whose commentary on my work has been exceedingly generous. They helped me find the right words, the right references, and the right reasons for writing to begin with. It has truly been a gift to be in conversation with them. I am also grateful to Dr. Natalie Alvarez, Dr. Hallie Marshall, and Dr. Kevin McNeilly, who generously offered to read my work during summer hours, and whose thorough and thoughtful feedback helped me approach the project with a renewed perspective.

I owe extraordinary gratitude to everyone in the Department of Theatre and Film at the University of British Columbia, for all the ways in which they guided me over the years: Cam Cronin, Dr. Siyuan Liu,

Dr. Hallie Marshall, Dr. Olivia Michiko Gagnon, Ian Patton, Andrea Rabinovitch, and Karen Tong.

Special thanks to Dr. Michael Everton, who cemented my complicated love for academia with his impassioned lectures. Thanks also to Dr. Peter Dickinson, who greatly influenced my transition from literature to performance.

Countless others have helped me get through this process in one piece. For guidance, reassurance, and gentle nudging, thank you to Hanyang Jiang, Yuning Liu, Claire Fogal, Dr. Andy Zuliani, Dr. Eury Chang, Dr. Jason Lieblang, Dr. Natalia Esling, Dr. Julia Henderson, and Dr. Katrina Dunn. Foremost among these kind-hearted souls is Dr. Nate Szymanski, who has demystified this whole process for me at every step of the way and shared in some of the best excursions. Finally, my greatest gratitude goes to Geoffrey Morrison for his generous, generative, and gentle editorial support. Without him, I would have always used three adjectives where one would suffice.

My previous work at UBC was facilitated by generous financial support from the Joseph-Armand Bombardier Canada Graduate Scholarship (SSHRC), UBC's Four Year Doctoral Fellowship, the Stuart Keate Scholarship, the Mr. and Mrs. G. E. Poole Award, the Errol Durbach Award, the Interdisciplinary Histories Research Cluster, and the Public Scholars Initiative, along with travel grants that allowed me to present my research at conferences. I am also thankful to *Capacious: Journal for Emerging Affect Inquiry* for publishing a version of the sixth chapter, "Notes on Mad Listening."

Last but never least: without my family behind me, there would be no text in front of you. I could not have come this far without them. Above all, my most heartfelt thanks goes to my partner, Elissa Hanson, to whom this book is dedicated.

Contents

CHAPTER 1

Introduction

In an 1892 medical dictionary, lexicographer John Marie Keating outlines a term dating to the mid-nineteenth century: "asylum ear" or "mad ear," otherwise known in the period as *haematoma auris*, or today's "cauliflower ear." He describes the condition as a "thickening of the upper part of the external ear, sometimes found in the insane" (129). This injury was frequently passed off as a naturally occurring symptom, said to develop spontaneously. However, in 1888, Samuel Sexton, a medical physician specializing in diseases of the ear, observed that "there may often be reasons for suppressing the truth; persons may desire to conceal the fact of blows having been administered" (132). The truth is that madpersons were often struck upon the side of the head by "impatient attendants," and thus it was typically the left ear that suffered ("Injuries" 289).[1] The idea of a "mad ear" gives historical context to the intersections between madness and audition, and the ways that medical authorities have literally shaped patients' listening by deforming the ear itself. At the same time, we also witness the process of pathologization, by which mad subjects have routinely been blamed for the iatrogenic symptoms of their own medical mistreatment.

In this book, I am interested in the auditory experiences of mad-identified subjects, both on and offstage, and the means by which artists represent, approximate, simulate, or otherwise depict non-normative modes of listening. Imagining for a moment that someone was to reenact

M. Tomkinson, *Sound and Sense in Contemporary Theatre*,
https://doi.org/10.1007/978-3-031-78034-9_1

the scenario described above: what would it mean to listen through an asylum ear? What would that sound like on stage, or on the radio, or in a pair of headphones? Throughout the following chapters, I hope to engage more closely with precisely these kinds of aesthetic choices, while also attending to the representational politics of reconstructing mad auralities in performance.

A quick web search will suffice to show that there is considerable research and popular commentary on mad sounds. Fascination with mad songs and mad speech has probably been present for as long as people have been singing and talking, though the mad genre has been especially popular since the beginning of the seventeenth century, when the English folk song "Tom o' Bedlam" was written and later performed and reproduced widely. A century and a half onward, Thomas Percy's *Reliques of Ancient English Poetry* (1765) contains six canonical mad songs, supposed to be performed by itinerant Bedlamites. Stereotypes of mad sound have remained relatively consistent over time, as evidenced by the presence of Ophelia's ballads among countless examples of the "Sanity Slippage Song" in the TV Tropes database.

Auditory images of madness are everywhere. As Anne Carson observes, "It is in large part according to the sounds people make that we judge them sane or insane" (119). We might think we know, for example, what an asylum sounds like from listening to *One Flew Over the Cuckoo's Nest* (1975), recalling Billy Bibbit's stutter, or perhaps from witnessing the film adaptation of *Marat/Sade* (1967), in which the patients of Charenton vocalize their madness in overly-familiar cadences. Though these performances have engendered a wide range of scholarly studies, there is a relative lack of research on mad aurality in the context of theatre. In broader terms, we have a general—if not stereotypical—sense of what madness *sounds* like, but less has been said about what madness *hears* and *listens* like. This is not to say, however, that the conversation is entirely absent, which would be to disregard the extensive work done by mad activists, especially those within the Hearing Voices Movement—an international community of service users and psychiatric survivors whose efforts have greatly reshaped and destigmatized public understanding of voice hearing (McCarthy-Jones, 90).

To the wider sound studies glossary, then, I would propose adding a new term: "mad listening." As I emphasize throughout my case studies, this term is not meant to essentialize madness, or listening, by grouping diverse auditory experiences under one concept.[2] Quite the opposite: the political gesture that my research initiates will, I hope, be a critical move towards more complex and heterogeneous listening experiences. For now, we can think of "mad listening" as a mad-positive orientation to sound, as well as a means to counter psychonormative assumptions about aurality. We might begin by asking: what kinds of listening go with the myriad varieties of madness? Or, put differently, what specific sounds are assigned to what specific mad aural experiences?

Given that these experiences are incredibly wide-ranging, this book narrows in on theatrical representations of mad aurality in a Western context, then zooms in a notch further on contemporary theatre and performance, where we will consider how madness is mediated within current cultural imaginaries by means of sound. As mad studies continues to grow as a discipline, it is necessary to trace its most urgent applications within today's artistic landscape, taking stock of persistent and pernicious assumptions before tracing these ideological presuppositions back to their sources, including those psychiatric institutions of the eighteenth century onward and the systems of thought that simultaneously bolstered them and emerged from them.

Were this a historical study, we could revisit Lope De Vega's *Madness in Valencia* (1590–1595) to find examples of characters diagnosing one another's madness through sound. We could also consider Chikamatsu Monzaemon's *The Love Suicides at Sonezaki* (1703) wherein a pair of suicidal lovers pause to listen to a temple bell. Or we might listen more closely to the final moments of August Strindberg's *Miss Julie* (1888), in which Jean, a servant, imagines that he hears a handbell ringing and cannot block out the sound. Indeed, bells that only the protagonist and audience can hear were central to Henry Irving's career success in his portrayal of guilty Mathias in *The Bells* (1871). Note that Ophelia also describes Hamlet's madness using bell imagery, suggesting that his "sovereign reason" is like "sweet bells jangled out of tune and harsh" (3.1.172). In the modernist period, Sophie Treadwell's *Machinal* (1928) is another potential case study for mad sound studies research, with its cacophonous opening scene featuring the sounds of "telephone bells, buzzers" and other mechanical devices signifying sonic oppression and alienation within the industrial era (1). Such audible imagery chimes with Dolly MacKinnon's study of early twentieth-century soundscapes within asylums. She writes, "According to the published memoirs of Margaret Isabel Wilson, who was institutionalized in America during the 1930s, 'There were bells, bells, bells; [and] orders, orders, orders' which governed every aspect of her life" (76). To isolate just one auditory stereotype here, the sound of bells is heavily associated with mad auralities across a variety of historical and cultural contexts, to the extent that this motif perhaps warrants its own study. For the most part, I leave this historical work to future scholars, and offer these chapters as a foundation for further inquiry in this subject area. To this end, I acknowledge that there is much work to be done, not only in bridging disciplines and recovering mad histories, but also in remapping this research beyond North America and Europe, where my current focus lies.[3]

In its emphasis on non-normative forms of listening, this study resonates with the aural diversity movement led by John Drever and Andrew Hugill. The Aural Diversity Network proceeds from the fact that there is a vast range of hearing differences, ranging from "traumas and shocks" to simply "having a cold," which can dramatically affect one's auditory perception (para. 3). In their edited collection, *Aural Diversity* (2022), Drever and Hugill ask an important question regarding hierarchies of hearing: namely, "whose ear has primacy in disciplines that are built on an assumption of otological normalcy?" ("Aural Diversity: Book" para. 3). Their work, and that of the book's contributors, seeks to challenge audism, auraltypicality, and other forms of discrimination against those with non-normative auditory perception. Bridging sound and psychology, Drever notes that "auraldiversity may intersect with someone's neurodiversity, such as the case of autism with hyperacute hearing" ("Primacy" 19). Thinking alongside this larger project, my hope is that this book will make an original contribution to this emerging conversation by integrating mad politics, methodologies, and lived experiences more fully into the theoretical paradigm of aural diversity, whose focus on neurodivergence is, as of yet, limited in scope.

Since the early aughts, a number of multidisciplinary scholars have considered the relationship between sound and madness, including Carolyn Birdsall, La Marr Jurelle Bruce, Simon Cross, Anja Drautzburg, Anna Harpin, Christopher Dingwall-Jones, Matt Selway, Nicola Shaughnessy, Senta Siewert, Jon Venn, Neil Verma, and Scott Wallin. An even smaller number have touched upon the aural dimension of mad representation and experience. To date, the scholarly approach of Birdsall and Siewert comes closest to my own. Their essay, "Of Sound Mind: Mental Distress and Sound in the Twentieth-Century Media Culture" (2013), lays some critical groundwork for this project. Identifying a gap in the literature, the authors note that sonic representations of madness have received minimal attention compared to Sander Gilman's foundational studies of visual representations of madness. Many of the initial impulses that echo throughout my research appear in the above essay's overview, which addresses an abundance of topics, including acousmatic sound, representational strategies, sound design techniques, feminist critiques, overlapping cultural histories of madness/media/medicine, pathologized forms of listening, auditory simulations of madness, technological developments, and more. In revisiting this essay, one particularly generative question for my purposes—and one that guides my close listening—is whether there exists a "formula for aligning or 'audiopositioning' listeners with protagonists" (34). Throughout my case studies, I repeatedly return to this problem, which I consider to be the main theoretical bugbear, and central research question, of this book: by what means do theatre practitioners attempt to simulate the aural subjectivity of madpersons? To my knowledge, this study is among the first to treat this desire for perceptual "alignment" as a problem. Where other scholars have broached this topic, there is a tendency to overemphasize the liberatory potential in this empathetic gesture, which is usually framed as a play on the old cliché: "to listen for a minute with someone else's ears."

Intersubjective listening—hearing another's hearing—is a worthy project, but I hope to outline some of the potential issues with "becoming other" through sonic empathy. Headphone theatre, for example, perpetuates this fantasy by allegedly recreating another person's point of audition inside one's own head. All too often, however, critics end up talking about the virtual as though it were actual, despite knowing the difference, because this act of ostensible mind-melding seems to serve the public good. On some occasions, however, what appears to be a more empathetic mode of listening may actually be just another form of fetishism, where audiences are promised a "mad experience" whose formal and ethical contours go unquestioned. On this front, Arielle Silverman cautions that disability simulations can have the unintended effect of amplifying "people's preexisting fears and misconceptions" (para. 8). Silverman adds that this practice is "highly controversial among disability activists," suggesting that "more research on this topic is badly needed" (para. 3). In line with this prompt, this book ultimately aims to trouble simulatory aesthetics, which in many cases serve to reinforce sanism, even when they appear under the guise of facilitating empathy and understanding. As such, my case studies take a more critical approach in unpacking the specific staging conventions of mad aural subjectivity, while querying what Ross Brown calls the "quasi-acoustic intracranial space" of the mind, in concert with sound's material, political, spatial, affective, and phenomenological inflections (73). In many ways, examining these inflections is more important than determining a simulation's efficacy, as Tanya Titchkosky, Devon Healey, and Rod Michalko remind us when they pose two crucial questions for our purposes—namely: "What sort of knowledge does simulation stimulate? What interests ground this way of knowing?" (123).

Pandemic Proviso

Perhaps I might speak more directly to what personal interests ground this research. Thinking back to December 2020, an article in the *Guardian* described the COVID-19 pandemic as the "greatest threat to mental health since the second world war" (para. 1). I would be remiss not to acknowledge the profound yet immeasurable effect that this situation had on me and my research at the time. In order to set the stage for the discussions that follow, allow me to share an illuminating anecdote: You may remember the "7 pm clap" for healthcare workers that persisted throughout the first year of the pandemic, when people would go to their windows with pots and pans to cheer on frontline workers. At first, this ritual had an uplifting effect on me. I eagerly poked my head outside and took solace in this act of sonic solidarity. Over time, however, this ritual turned into a routine and eventually became something of a reflex. Upon hearing the first few claps, I would feel obligated to stand up and make my way to the window to perform my civic duty with a series of rehearsed gestures. In my experience of so-called obsessive–compulsive disorder, these kinds of repetitive behaviours can quickly take on a distressing aspect, even if the activity is benign—and this is precisely what happened with the "7 pm clap," which became, for me, a compulsory action. Clouded by superstition, a small part of me believed that if I did not participate in the clapping, then I or someone I care about would get sick and die. Most evenings, in the lead-up to the applause, my eyes were fixed on the clock, my ears and hands primed. I set alarms to make sure I would not miss a day. Even if I was preoccupied with cooking or cleaning, I would take a second to put my hands together a few times in a small golf clap, just to be sure I had made the gesture. Not to belabour the point, but you can see why the topic of mad listening has had such personal resonance for me, and the extent to which the present book operates methodologically on the same plane that it studies. This will become especially clear in my sixth chapter, where I share more examples from my lived experience, in order to claim value for mad epistemologies within the production and transmission of academic knowledge.

Mad Methodologies

By surveying various permutations of simulated madness in contemporary theatre and performance, I attempt to define the fuzzy boundaries of this model I call mad auralities. Drawing inspiration from Sara Ahmed, I treat this concept as an orientation and a theoretical site of encounter, rather than a prescriptive category (5). There are three general courses of intervention throughout this book. The first entails close listening to theatrical case studies in order to discern their representational strategies, dispute phoney phenomenologies, and demonstrate the cultural impact of these plays' approaches to aural dramaturgy. On this front, I also attend to the critical reception of the productions in question, addressing common assumptions and ellipses around shared auralities, while urging more caution around claims for the power of simulation to promote intersubjective empathy. Indeed, at times this book more closely resembles discourse analysis than theatre theory, insofar as I am interested in the ways that people talk about mad auralities, including the kinds of metaphors they use, and the role that this phenomenon plays in different conversations, both publicly and academically. In some sense, the plays at the centre of each chapter are vehicles for a larger theoretical engagement with representational problematics. The book's second critical axis entails the development of a fragmentary topography of mad auralities based on my lived experience, as presented in the sixth chapter. Finally, my third intervention concerns mad listening as an interpretive framework, an attempt on my part to write, listen, and reason madly during the composition of these chapters.

My own multipronged approach to this study draws precedent from books such as Andrew Sofer's *Dark Matter: Invisibility in Drama, Theater, and Performance* (2013). In this book, he identifies four domains—practical, historical, aesthetic, and ideological—within which to identify and grapple with scholarly issues (11). My guiding research questions broadly centre around each of these areas, though I do not always maintain an equal balance between them. In its simplest iteration, my overarching research question concerns the practical: How have contemporary theatre practitioners staged mad auralities? Next, there is the historical: Do we find any continuities in what a mad point of audition sounds like over time? Considering that this is partly a question of representational strategies, we might ask: What kinds of aesthetic conventions underlie popular representations of mad auralities? Finally, in the realm of ideology, I ask: How do these artists work towards combating stereotypes and rewriting cultural scripts around mad representation, or, conversely, how do they perpetuate harmful understandings of mad aurality by way of essentialization, medicalization, and other means of reification? In asking these questions, I share Sofer's plainly stated research objective to locate representational issues that "might otherwise evade detection" (12).

My research focuses on contemporary drama with a North American and European reach, moving geographically between Canada, England, Germany, and the United States. I have chosen these plays in particular because they are, for the most part, popular or canonical works that have a relatively wide public reception and that epitomize many of the sonic conventions I focus upon here. As such, they represent a solid foundation on which to build future research. Despite their popularity, I have also chosen these works because they have not yet been studied very thoroughly. Moreover, their respective formal innovations offer multiple points of access into sonic representations of madness. Though my case studies are primarily critical and do not focus on many mad-identified artists, I hope to fulfil that role myself in the sixth chapter, which centres my own lived experience.

Invoking a co-constitutive model of madness, Drew Daniel argues that such experiences are not just internal, but also interpretive—"not just a feeling but a claim about the feeling, a socially extended assemblage composed out of consciousness, expression, a regime of knowledge, and at least one body" (27). Similarly, I map madness as an emergent phenomenon, irreducible to any one person's life world or diagnosis, though fully respecting these personal truths. Pursuing the concept of emergence further, this study follows ostensibly unsound methodological principles, foregoing a one-size-fits-all interpretive method for a noisy intersection of theoretical approaches. One justification for this approach comes from Daniel, who suggests that the "estranging, disorganizing power" of madness should be matched by a "polychronic assemblage" of critical materials (31). In constellating three main fields—mad studies, sound studies, and theatre studies —there are indeed many mixed methodologies for which to account.

From a mad studies perspective—citing scholars such as Brenda LeFrançois, Richard Ingram, Anna Harpin, Ken Gale, Peter Beresford, Petra Kuppers, Robert McRuer, Johanna Braun, La Marr Jurelle Bruce, Therí Alyce Pickens, and many others—I draw upon a heterogeneous ensemble of theoretical tools and praxes. Following Bruce in particular, who characterizes "mad methodology as a parapositivist approach insofar as it resists the hegemony of positivism," I take a critical stance towards the medicalization and pathologization of madness (10). In this regard, I extend what Bruce calls "radical compassion" towards madpersons, in validating non-normative epistemologies and taking seriously any claim that others might call "delusional" (10). At the same time, Bruce reminds us that radical compassion must involve a degree of critical ambivalence: that is, we must hold liberatory potential and hegemonic harm in tension, even when they show up in the same person, place, or representational structure" (9). To this end, my case studies offer both critical close listening and reparative work, attempting to balance the two approaches by means of formal description and explication. In other words, throughout this book, I am primarily interested in figuring out precisely how these works signify and aestheticize madness. That said, I also recognize the importance of addressing the potential representational harms perpetuated through tropes, stereotypes, clichés, and so on—and I do not shy away from pointed critique of these features where necessary. Playing to the middle is not an inherently productive scholarly approach, however, and ambivalence has its critics. William Cheng, for example, has suggested that "ambivalence feels responsible and, for all its virtuosity, sounds humble" (46), and yet "distractions may be partly responsible for how sonic offenses go unaddressed" (33). To me, a simple solution entails approaching ambivalence from both standpoints rather than neither—whether critical, suspicious, paranoid, deconstructive, or reparative, generative, counterintuitive, and weak.[4] According to Cheng, "weak critical modes" (16) like the reparative will "dare to be fallible" (40). Along similar lines, Jonathan Sterne, in his book *Diminished Faculties: A Political Phenomenology of Impairment* (2021), describes "impairment phenomenology" as being "different from other kinds of phenomenology in that it does not assume a subject in command of their own faculties" (12). Following this thread further, Sterne bolsters one of the central theses of this book when he writes that "One of the ironic results of disability simulations is that they produce too much stability in accounts of experience—'this is how it really works'—because they have not spent enough time to acquire the variety of experiences that come from living with an impairment or disability. A political phenomenology of impairment should be more unstable, because it takes more time; and while it may traffic in hypotheses and fictions, those are generated from real conditions of impairment" (14).

A mad studies project, by any conscientious standards, "must be empirically incomplete and inadequate to the plurality of experience," just as Sterne describes his own project (14). In one regard, then, I wish to challenge hegemonic forms of academic knowledge production by relinquishing any authority that comes from a false sense of scholarly empiricism—or, as Bruce puts it, to "deviate from the logics of positivism" (10). Moreover, I hope to put into practice Mel Y. Chen's observation that "partial knowing" can work "agonistically against and thus also with comprehension" (182).

These ideas come to a head in my sixth chapter, which explores autotheory as an alternative approach to standard academic research. In her research on the history and growing popularity of autotheory, Lauren Fournier describes the practice as both "theory and performance, autobiography and philosophy, research and creation" (40). Importantly, Fournier also stresses the intersectionality of autotheory:

> It is a term that describes a self-conscious way of engaging with theory – as a discourse, frame, or mode of thinking and practice – alongside lived experience and subjective embodiment, something very much in the *Zeitgeist* of cultural production today – especially in feminist, queer, and BIPOC – Black, Indigenous, and people of color – spaces that live on the edges of art and academia. (18)

My own intersections are these: I am a white settler scholar who identifies as mad and genderqueer. Appropriately, I would stress that this book—and especially my autotheoretical writing—only speaks to my own highly partial interpretive experience, and although I aim to incorporate a plurality of critical voices in my work, I cannot claim to speak as one for the many. Nonetheless, Fournier reminds us that "The singular can be a gateway to the multiple. And in theorizing together we may, after all, hear ourselves" (319). In this way, I consider this research to be a means of adding my voice to the mad movement at large, rather than an impossible distillation of mad thought across numerous cultural contexts.

Concerning sonic methodologies applied in a theatrical context, I ultimately move alongside Cheng in "listening for better worlds" (10). My research engages in conversation with a wide array of sound scholars who have imagined their own versions including Brian Kane, Brandon LaBelle, William Cheng, Ross Brown, Adrian Curtin, Lynne Kendrick, Mladen Ovadija, Salomé Voegelin, Marie Thompson, Dylan Robinson, François J. Bonnet, Jonathan Sterne, Jennifer Lynn Stoever, Fred Moten, Jean-Luc Nancy, and many others, who I will engage with in turn throughout the case studies that follow.

As Marcel Cobussen declares in the introduction to *The Bloomsbury Handbook of Sonic Methodologies* (2021), co-authored with Michael Bull, "I always search for a methodology that is responsive, responsible, and attentive to the specificity of the sonic material under investigation" (9). With this in mind, I do not subscribe to any single hermeneutical approach; rather, I try to approach my case studies with a plurality of interpretive strategies that span a material-discursive spectrum.[5] Most reliably, my case studies take a familiar scholarly approach in close listening to representational techniques in order to glean their formal, aesthetic, and cultural functions. Notwithstanding the audist assumptions present in the following quote, Anette Hoffmann defines close listening as "the attempt to know by ear, that is, to grasp as much as possible of the audible features of a recording" (534).[6] After Eve Kosofsky Sedgwick, scholars such as William Cheng have discouraged "paranoid" reading as the default academic impulse. Paranoid readings, according to Cheng, are built upon notions of authority, hierarchy, ambition, suspicion, deconstruction, cynicism, negative affect, self-satisfaction, and self-evident truths (4). Rather than abandoning paranoid reading and defecting to the reparative mode—pathologizing madness in the process—we should instead recuperate paranoia as a good-faith interpretive strategy. Can we listen closely and critically, I wonder, without listening adversarially? In the following chapters, I have tried my best to apply this question.

Another key methodological prong at play here belongs to theatre and performance studies. On this front, I am particularly indebted to George Home-Cook's "phenomenological consideration of theatrical listening" in *Theatre and Aural Attention: Stretching Ourselves* (2015). Home-Cook defines theatrical listening in the following terms: first, it involves "paying attention to atmospheres" (3); second, it relies on a combination of senses (4); and third, it is shaped by specific subjective and cultural contexts (10). Like Home-Cook, I proceed from sense experience towards close analysis, in awareness that reception starts with perception. Glancing back at the title of this book, one might triple underline "sense" as a keyword with multiple valences in my usage, ranging from sensibility to sensicality.

Most if not all of the sounds that I encountered throughout the course of this research took the form of archival recordings, which I accessed online and listened to through a set of Beyerdynamic DT 770 headphones. As "dynamic" as this device may be, it is not a perfect substitute for live attendance. At the same time, headphones encourage a kind of ethos of objectivity that can occasionally feel at odds with an anti-positivist approach, in light of various forensic techniques such as rewinding, slowing down, looping, boosting volume, and more. To some extent, this approach was born of necessity because of the vagaries of writing amid a global pandemic, which meant very few opportunities to attend live performances. At the risk of raising the spectre of liveness (namely, the question of whether I have experienced the *real* plays), I have decided to leave this conundrum intact by presenting this book in its pandemic form, true to the modes of engagement that were available to me at that time.

In another light, from an access perspective, this study has clearly benefited from the ability to listen more deliberately, with extensive control over playback. In *Hungry Listening: Resonant Theory for Indigenous Sound Studies* (2020), Dylan Robinson asks: "Is it even possible to have one ear open to the unknown and another to one's positionality? To what extent does this simply result in a kind of "schizo-audition" that forecloses upon Deep Listening?" (249). Though I am apprehensive to adopt the language of pathology here, I find that archival audio offers the possibility to do both of the things that Robinson describes—to listen multiple times with a different point of focus, and in the process critically examine the relationship between sound and self.

Drawing further inspiration from Sofer's working model, my chapters serve as independent, standalone case studies, because this allows me to focus on specific problems that arise in different performance contexts, where the "theoretical and methodological terms are set by the issue at hand" (16). My second chapter narrows in on acousmatic sound, for example, while the fourth centres on feminist theatrical adaptations, the fifth concerns the intersection between anti-Black and antimad ideology, and the sixth employs autotheory to explore mad listening from the inside out. These represent a few distinct sites of mad aural representation, where close analysis affords the opportunity to resist sanism and combat stigma—two of this study's foremost aims. To this end, my second chapter considers *The Eradication of Schizophrenia in Western Lapland* (2014) by Ridiculusmus; the fourth chapter considers *Ophelia's Zimmer* (2015) by Katie Mitchell and *Her Long Black Hair* (2004) by Janet Cardiff; the fifth chapter considers *Here are the Fragments* (2019) by Suvendrini Lena; and, finally, the sixth chapter is an autoethnographic study with an audio component. This final chapter stands apart from the rest in employing arts-based research methods, with the support of UBC's Public Scholars Initiative (PSI), which provides resources to students who wish to expand the horizons of their work through non-traditional formats (in my case, an audio essay, which can be found in *Capacious: Journal for Emerging Affect Inquiry*, Vol. 3, No.1).

Mad Auralities in Popular Culture

At the same cultural moment when the COVID-19 pandemic had been deemed a mental health crisis, Warner Bros. premiered the *Arkham Asylum Immersive Experience* in London in September, 2022: "Set in a vast, multi-sensory recreation of the psychiatric hospital, Arkham Asylum will be an epic alternate reality, combining futuristic technology and interactive theatrics with a wholly original story to create an unforgettable experience. Audiences are invited to lose themselves in the infamous asylum" ("Arkham" n.pag). There is something of a contemporary theatrical obsession with the "immersive asylum," and this production is just one of many, including *One Flew Over the Cuckoo's Nest: An Immersive Experience* (2018) by After Hours Theatre Company, and *Then She Fell* (2012) by Third Rail Projects, which was performed exactly 4,444 times in New York over the span of seven years. On a much larger scale, Broadway productions such *Next to Normal* (2008), *The Curious Incident of the Dog in the Night-Time* (2012), *Dear Evan Hansen* (2015), and *Be More Chill* (2015) have set in motion a wave of mental health conversations in the public sphere, for better or worse. Noting the popularity of these productions, it is clear that the social impact of mad representations is not simply relegated to mainstream TV and film, but also pervades the experience economy via theatre.[7] The plays at the centre of my case studies are nowhere near the scale of the megahit, but they still have considerable cultural reach, and thus a profound ability to shape how madness is understood. Having published elsewhere on some of the mainstream productions mentioned above, this study turns instead towards smaller-scale works on the fringes, which present a degree of nuance not always found on larger stages. As the editors of *Mad Matters: A Critical Reader in Canadian Mad Studies* (2013) note, the discipline "will have little meaning if it cannot offer some sense of an alternative" (18). As such, I proceed from the relatively less familiar towards the familiar, with the hope that this research might serve as a reference point for broader cultural criticism around mad aesthetics.

According to Sander Gilman, "Western culture understands disease, even mental illness, in aesthetic terms" (*Disease and Representation* 231). Stereotypical madness representations are pervasive and persistent in popular culture, including the Broadway productions mentioned above, but we also find harmful aesthetic conventions in local experimental theatre. I am especially interested in noting where performance ethics and aesthetics are misaligned, as in Anna Harpin's study of Katie Mitchell's "forensic" theatrical aesthetics (discussed further in Chapter 4), which she rightly claims are counterproductive to mad-positive and feminist representation. As Gilman's research indicates, aesthetics have both a positive and negative pole, along which are situated different representations of madness. In *Disability Aesthetics* (2010), Tobin Siebers suggests that disability can be a "critical framework for questioning aesthetic presuppositions in the history of art" (71). Drawing upon a definition of aesthetics put forward by eighteenth-century German philosopher Alexander Baumgarten, Siebers suggests that "aesthetics tracks the sensations that some bodies feel in the presence of other bodies"—whether curiosity, disgust, sympathy, or any range of feelings (1). One of the predominating aesthetic sensibilities of my four case studies is that of sonic empathy: the way that certain sounds can give someone the experience of hearing the world differently, from another person's subjective position. In this regard, one might say that this book concerns the aesthetics of simulation. Moreover, the question of representational ethics is inextricably intertwined with the formal strategies that theatre artists use to portray madness. The plays I discuss all participate in the social construction of madness as an aesthetic category, but, more than that, they partake in the taxonomizing and pathologizing of lived experiences that are categorized in the psy-sciences as disorders, e.g., "schizophrenia" as opposed to voice hearing. Ian Hacking states, with effective brevity, the consequences of typecasting: "Classification as schizophrenic affects the sensibilities of those classified"

(*Social Construction* 113). In this regard, aesthetic choices can be validating or invalidating, helpful or harmful, to the project of mad liberation. Though the aesthetics of simulation have generally been taken up with good intentions, my case studies demonstrate that the practice carries unintended risks and consequences, including an inadvertent deepening of binaries—sane and mad, us and them—that such simulations are often intended to unsettle.

Lineages of Mad Listening

Mad studies has undergone a growth spurt over the past decade as it continues to find purchase in a wide variety of contexts, from social work to prison abolition to live performance. As late as 2019, scholars such as Helen Spandler and Dina Poursanidou have called mad studies "an emerging new critical project," though it has been suspended in a state of newness for at least a decade, if not considerably longer when one broadens the definition (1). Richard Ingram, who coined the disciplinary term in 2008, suggests that scholars should not look outside-in at madness but instead use madness to assess the world—or, in other words: "If mad studies achieves its objectives, it needs to have as part of its end goal the shaking up, the disturbing, of all forms of academic knowledge [...] In short, could we perform making (non)sense together?" ("Doing Mad Studies" 14). From this quote, it is clear that mad methodologies have had a performative component since their inception, though of course such methodologies were practised long before they were labelled.[8] From the outset, mad studies has been a highly intersectional movement, operating in solidarity with "survivors of racism, colonialism, patriarchy, ableism, and related forms of material and cultural oppression" (LeFrançois et al. 19).

Among recent contributions to the field, La Marr Jurelle Bruce's *How to Go Mad without Losing Your Mind: Madness and Black Radical Creativity* (2021) is most notable.[9] Bruce's book is among the first in-depth examinations of madness in the context of Black radical theory and praxis. In redefining the field, Bruce also offers explicit models for theorizing madness, which have generally remained implicit until now. These include "phenomenal madness" (6), "medicalized madness" (7), and "psychosocial madness" (8), all of which represent different aspects of lived experience. The first concerns "unruliness of mind" and "crises of perception" (6); the second concerns "psychopathologies codified by the psy sciences of psychiatry" (7); and the third concerns "radical deviation from the normal within a given psychosocial milieu" (8). No doubt, the varieties of mad experience are not limited to these three categories, though they cover significant ground.[10]

I am principally indebted to Bruce's articulation of mad methodology, which is among the most concise and practical expressions of madness as a critical framework. Crucially, Bruce also emphasizes the aural dimension of madness, which sets up a number of conversations in this study. He writes:

> Mad methodology seeks, follows, and rides the unruly movements of madness. It reads and hears *idioms of madness*: those purported rants, raves, rambles, outbursts, mumbles, stammers, slurs, gibberish sounds, and unseemly silences that defy the grammars of Reason [...] Whereas rationalism roundly discredits madpersons, mad methodology recognizes madpersons as critical theorists and decisive protagonists in struggles for liberation. (9)

Following Bruce, my chapters are attuned to mad methodology as a listening practice. Taking this a step further, however, I am not simply invested in deciphering mad idioms; equally important to this study are the formal contexts and conceits inside of which listeners do such interpretive work. And yet, despite the promise and potential of a mad listening methodology, a sudden shift towards the sense of hearing, and away from ocularcentrism, should not be regarded as inherently productive—nor is a sensory binary itself productive, since the senses do not operate in isolation. As Therí Alyce Pickens notes, "the sonic confuses just as much as the ocular" (70). Accordingly, it is good to be suspicious about claims for sound's liberatory potential, which are all too easy to reiterate uncritically. Indeed, the majority of the following chapters are concerned with instances where such inflated claims are put to the test. Pickens adds that, just like the visual, the aural "opens up the possibilities for (mis)interpretation" (70). However, there is also emancipatory potential in sound that cannot be ignored, especially for subjects engaged in asymmetrical relations of power.

In theorizing "mad auralities," both words in my usage are historically and qualitatively freighted. It may be helpful, then, to parse them individually first, before considering some of the ways in which these concepts overlap. To start with the "mad," I concur with Bruce in treating madness as a "floating signifier," which ranges from unruly phenomenology to psychiatric pathology to states of anger and rage, or any sense of difference experienced as a result of living within a psychonormative society (8). By mobilizing this term, I work towards centring people with lived experience, combating stereotypes, holding space for irrationality and unreason, troubling psychiatric discourse, and celebrating Mad Pride.

Though the term "mad" is not without its opponents, my decision to use this theoretical framework follows from a number of well-respected scholars in the field: "As with queer," writes Margaret Price in her landmark book *Mad at School* (2011), "the broad scope of mad carries the drawback of generality but also the power of mass" (10). As a believer in critical tension, I do not negate the value of psychiatric labels and adapt my terminology to suit specific contexts—especially those in which a person has expressed a personal preference for medical language, or requires such a vocabulary to navigate the healthcare industry or legitimize a medical leave.

Shifting focus to the second term in my title, "auralities," we might immediately question its audist connotations, given the word's etymological origin in the Latin *auris* or "ear." Along these lines, Seth Kim-Cohen, in his book *In the Blink of an Ear* (2009) proposes a "non-cochlear sound art" (2009). As Christoph Cox puts it in his review, such art becomes "non-cochlear" when it abandons its "aural fixation" and "leaps across the differences between ear, eye, and hand" ("Artforum" n.pag). Linking mad praxis to other intersections of radical unreasoning, this study presents similar challenges to audist and phonocentric assumptions, which tend to abound where listening subjectivities are concerned. This is especially true of my sixth chapter, where I outline some of my own attempts at non-cochlear listening, with reference to notable sound work by Deaf artists. These intersections are important, not least of all because they prevent "mad auralities" from becoming essentialized and fixating too intently on the aural.[11] There are reasons not to abandon the word "aurality" entirely, however. In my case, I prefer the word for its potential meanings in the plural, in ways that "listenings" does not quite capture. And though it is rooted in the "ear," I take this to mean any organ of listening, whether skin or skull or spine—though we are also not limited to physiology, and can imagine speculative, non-human ears just the same. In *Aurality: Listening and Knowledge in Nineteenth-Century Colombia* (2014), Ana María Ochoa Gautier notes that the ear "seems to lie ambiguously between physiology and physics," but, yet again, the ambiguities do not have to stop here (208).[12]

One of the central philosophical tensions in this book concerns the gap between exceptionality and commonality, universalism and individualism. In *The Order of Sounds: A Sonorous Archipelago* (2016), Robin Mackay writes that "the potential for extravagant delirium is constitutive of the basic mechanisms of cognitive synthesis" (19). Drawing on the nineteenth-century historian Hippolyte Taine, Mackay argues that hallucination, for example, could be considered "the basic fact of mental life" (12). Though I try to maintain epistemological tension in the case studies that follow, I am careful to not simply honour lived experience through essentialization, or to normalize madness through universalization. At the same time, my research approaches mad representations with a critical ear, questioning their formal relationship to firsthand experiences of mad aurality—and, in some unavoidable ways, measuring the distance. Meanwhile, the above-mentioned concept of aural diversity exposes the fiction of universals, whether mad, sane, both, or neither. It even calls into question the biological basis of Mackay's "basic mechanisms." By investing in this concept, the shift towards radical individuation among listeners is a timely and appropriate response to much sound studies research, which has tended to imagine an ideal or transcendental listener situated at an Archimedean point.

Staging Intersubjectivity

Though many critical analyses in theatre studies involve an element of listening to performance, relatively few are concerned with performances of listening. Anna Harpin's work in *Madness, Art, and Society: Beyond Illness* (2018) is a notable exception, wherein she attends to the ways in which characters listen, and how their listening is represented formally. Harpin seeks out moments, for example, when the audience is invited to "look and listen with, not at" a mad character (28). Her earlier collection, *Performance and Participation: Practices, Audiences, Politics* (2016), co-edited with Helen Nicholson, includes an essay by Deirdre Heddon, who formalizes this idea of *withness* as "entangled listening" (19). Heddon defines this process as one of "listening out for listening" or "stretching towards" meaning (23). There is, as one might expect, a strong ethical component to the author's sense of entanglement, which is rooted in Jean-Luc Nancy's philosophical project of ontological co-existence—in the sense that one is always intersubjectively entangled with other people (28). This further relates to Luce Irgaray's notion of ethical listening as an act of "being with" which requires that one not "subject difference to sameness and similarity" (118).

Applying this philosophy to a theatrical context, Harpin makes strong claims for intersubjectivity in her chapter "Figuring Perceptual Experiences on Stage and Screen," where she writes: "As an audience we temporarily cohabit the internal landscape of Stuart's imagination [...] In effect, instead of watching the duck glide across the water, we are dunked underwater so we can see the flippers frantically paddling beneath" (113). If Harpin starts with this premise, however, she ultimately comes to the opposite conclusion in arguing for "an ethical practice of care based on difference and not knowing" or, in other words, "empathy without sameness" (103). Contrary to an ethics of intersubjectivity predicated on shared experiences, Harpin reminds us that theatre always contains a multiplicitous reality. In the introductory chapter to an earlier collection, *Performance, Madness, and Psychiatry: Isolated Acts* (2014), the author examines how theatre makers toy with "the tyranny of normative, consensus reality" in constructing perceptual experiences (12). For my part, I am interested in how theatre makers inadvertently craft new consensus realities, even as they attempt to escape the normative—for example, treating all manifestations of madness the same way, or imagining the audience as a hive mind.

Here, Harpin makes an extremely crucial point for the purposes of this book. Specifically, she suggests that realism, as a theatrical approach to representing madness accurately, only "tends to remainder the contents of 'mad' experience in some ways as outside the dramatic frame and, thereby, implicitly participates in an othering of such states of mind" (189). She continues:

> Madness in such works is, frequently, reduced to identifiable surface behaviours that are framed as 'ill', behaviours that exceed the limits of the internal logic of the play-world. From Christopher's blue oranges to Ophelia's unbound hair and wild song to Blanche Du Bois's terrors, cries and scratches, madness is frequently lurid. As Darian Leader notes, madness is also commonly culturally framed as spectacular in so far as it is so often 'so visible, so tangible, so audible'. Madness is often, then, excessive action or difference witnessed by the stage sane. (189)

Throughout her scholarly oeuvre, Harpin takes a consistent position—namely, that mad metaphors are best when they are ambiguous and not lurid, such as Sarah Kane's use of light and mirrors to "rehabilitate and complicate" tropes that equate madness with darkness (189).[13] Through complicating such tropes, Harpin hopes that mad-positive stagings can help take audiences "round the bend, not to have a pseudo-experience of madness; but rather to have an encounter that softens the false distinctions between us and them" (188). Following Harpin, I take a similar approach in focusing intently on pseudo-experiences of madness (i.e., approximations and simulations) and the formal means by which they are generated through sound. My research in subsequent chapters reveals the extent to which such staged encounters—often predicated on phoney phenomenologies of madness—tend to harden, as opposed to soften, false distinctions between self and other.

Between Harpin and Heddon there is a shared desire to construe listening as an ethical act of connection between bodyminds, whether through "withness" or "entanglement." Furthermore, these ideas call to mind Jean-Luc Nancy's writing on resonance, which is well-cited by scholars situated at the intersection of theatre and sound studies. Among them, George Home-Cook is perhaps most in touch with Nancy's theatricality. In *Theatre and Aural Attention: Stretching Ourselves* (2015), he responds to Nancy's question of "What is at play in listening?" by saying that "there is indeed much 'at play' in listening" since it is "in every sense, an act: listening is not only something that we do, but is inherently *theatrical*" (9). Its performativity derives from the fact that perception is always "unfinished, ephemeral, and in process" (8).

Setting the stage for Home-Cook, Nancy's *Listening* (2009) argues that listening is an act of aural stretching (*tendre l'oreille*) towards the thing being listened to. This notion of stretching towards understanding places less emphasis on deciphering a sound's composition, and more on feeling its resonances. Indeed, his concept of the "diapason-subject" compares subjectivity to a tuning fork. In his review of Nancy's book, Michael Gallope clarifies the philosopher's distinction between hearing and listening as such: "Where *entendre* [hearing] implies the closure of understanding and truth, *ecouter* [listening] implies the openness of negotiation, uncertainty, and exposure" (158). Already, one can see how Nancy's suspicion towards pre-encoded signification might be useful for a mad project such as this one, which is interested in sounds on the "edge of meaning" (*Listening* 7). In preserving a sense of anti-closure and non-indexicality, Nancy's concept of listening is another useful touchstone for this study. If it is true that we, as listeners, do not simply "receive a communicated meaning that awaits us," then auditory simulations are inherently compromised in their quest for reproducing experiences (158). Throughout my case studies, I share Gallope's position that "we cannot fuse our nervous systems together in a perfect solidarity, nor can we communicate information among one another without remainder, distortion, or excess" (159). In many ways, my approach is one of noticing and describing these remainders.

In his book Hungry Listening: Resonant Theory for Indigenous Sound Studies (2020), Dylan Robinson marks a profound discrepancy between colonial and anti-colonial ways of listening, most notably in "encounters between Indigenous song and Western art music" (1). In writing about Indigenous epistemologies, Robinson troubles the "whiteness of sound studies" and redresses a lack of research on decolonial listening practices in a Canadian context (37). The title phrase, "hungry listening," describes an explicitly settler colonial form of perception. According to Robinson, "it is a 'civilizing' sensory paradigm that has been imposed on Indigenous people who grew up within residential school, boarding school, and day school systems [...]" (3). The author describes the function of Indigenous songs as being multiplicitous in ways that settler colonial listening practices fail to acknowledge and thus tend to flatten. Indigenous song, he says, expresses not only musical content, but also law and history, whereas these subjects are typically limited to written communication in Western traditions (46). When Indigenous songs are colonized in the process of mishearing, says Robinson, they are subjected to "epistemic violence" (46). Robinson broadly defines decolonial listening in terms of productive ambiguity, multi-sense engagement, and resisting the "hunger" of the book's title to "consume alterity" (72). Settler colonial listening practices reflect a civilizing drive, where listeners are expected to sit still and practice calm aesthetic appreciation. Unsettling listening, then, means acknowledging our own perceptual frameworks as listeners.

Most helpful to my research are Robinson's comments on critical listening positionality. "As part of our listening positionality," writes Robinson, "we each carry listening privilege, listening biases, and listening ability that are never wholly positive or negative; by becoming aware of normative listening habits and abilities, we are better able to listen otherwise" (10). However, Robinson suggests that in challenging normative ways of listening, we should not simply pivot to Indigenous modes of engagement, because this "might result in an auditory form of 'going native'" (247). The author also draws a helpful distinction between identity and positionality, suggesting that the latter is shiftier and changes based on the cultural context of one's listening, as well as one's relation to the space or land that one occupies at the time of listening. Each of my chapters is informed by Robinson's prompt to attend to privileges and biases, and, on this front, I aim to be as transparent as possible about my own listening positionality as a white settler scholar. In consonance with Robinson's concerns about perceptual forms of "going native," this dissertation is similarly concerned with auditory forms of "cripping up" or what I call "factitious listening," which I use to refer to instances where actors, critics, playwrights, or audience members feign or mimic the aural symptomatology of a specific condition. Kaite O'Reilly popularized the term "cripping up," which is widely used in disability studies to refer to non-disabled actors playing disabled roles. At the same time, Ellen Samuels, in *Fantasies of Identification: Disability, Gender, Race* (2014) cautions against gatekeeping disability by trying to parse "real" identities from "fake" ones. While I concur with Samuels that we must grant "greater authority to the expert knowledge that individuals have about their own bodies" (214), I also share La Marr Jurelle Bruce's concern that "to walk a mile in someone else's shoes and amble, like a tourist, through their lifeworld" has the potential to leave those with lived experience "existentially barefoot all the while" (10).

Encapsulating one of my central preoccupations as a mad-identified scholar, Robinson proposes a form of listening that "does not reduce what is heard to the knowable" and that "understands sound in its irreducible alterity" (64). Proposing an alternative phenomenology of listening, Robinson references the classical composer Helmut Lachenmann, who suggests "observing an acoustic event from the perspective of 'What happened?'" as opposed to mining its significance (249). To this end, my case studies take up a quasi-descriptive mode, explicating formal devices rather than mounting evidence for a devastating critique. Indeed, I return often to Bruce's concept of "critical ambivalence," which reckons with "the simultaneous harm and benefit" of mad representations (242). This strikes me as a novel position for scholarly criticism, and one that is best suited to the topic at hand, which is rife with ambiguities and tensions.

Chapter Overview

In the next chapter, I examine a play which has attracted many dubious claims: *The Eradication of Schizophrenia in Western Lapland* (2014) by Jon Haynes and David Woods of Ridiculusmus. The play's official writeup describes "an audience split in two experiencing auditory hallucinations" (para. 1). Along the same lines, reviewers such as Laura Barnett in the *Guardian* have said that the show "replicates the experience of having an auditory hallucination" (para. 1). To this end, the play features a dividing wall that separates the stage into two sides, with the audience sitting on one side and "hearing voices" from beyond the wall. Taking this claim to its furthest conclusion, another writeup on the company's website says that this "innovative staging offers visitors a unique and three-dimensional insight into what it is to be psychotic" ("Shows in Rep"). In this chapter, I consider the formal, phenomenological, and rhetorical dimensions of mad auditory simulation, focusing on the aforementioned metaphor of "replication." As Brian Kane writes in *Sound Unseen: Acousmatic Sound in Theory and Practice* (2014): "One central, replicated feature of acousmatic listening appears to be that under-determination of the sonic source encourages imaginative supplementation" (9). Kane adds that acousmatic listening—cutting off sounds from their visual sources—has often been used to give audiences a sense of the transcendental, including a sense of others' interiority (9). On this point, I question the tendency of critics to downplay the metaphoricity of acousmatic listening in service of a fantasy of aural intersubjectivity. Moreover, the idea that sharing a facsimile of auditory hallucinations can convey the experience of voice hearing fails to locate so-called mental illness beyond the mind. What are the consequences, then, of forgetting the "as if" of affective experiences? Or can we ignore such disavowals for the sake of the greater good: identification, empathy, and understanding? Noting Kane's description of the Pythagorean veil as a "screen of fetishism"—a screen behind which the philosopher was said to lecture—I am mindful of the literal screen that sits in the middle of this production and, accordingly, I interrogate the role it plays in the aesthetics and ethics of aural simulation (211).

In the book's third chapter, I offer a comparative analysis of two immersive performances that offer different representations of the "madwoman," and which use different technological means to portray their protagonists' subjective listening positions. One of these two case studies shifts locales to a recent play at the Schaubühne theatre in Berlin: Alice

Birch and Katie Mitchell's *Ophelia's Zimmer* (2015), a recent adaptation of *Hamlet* which depicts the offstage events leading up to Ophelia's death, set within a prison-like bedroom that slowly fills up with water and is eventually enclosed in a large plexiglass box. The show uses traditional Foley techniques, featuring an enclosed room upstage where cast members create sound effects and throw their voices. In adapting *Hamlet*, the show moves away from text and towards the aural in some other important ways. Letters to Ophelia, for example, are delivered to her room in cassette form and played over a vintage cassette player. With reference to Bridget Escolme's essay "Ophelia Confined: Madness and Infantilization in Some Versions of *Hamlet*" (2014), I suggest that the protagonist is confined not just spatially, but aurally. Drowned in a sound world beyond her creation—and crafted offstage by men—we see Ophelia at the centre of various sonic forms of control. Escolme suggests that while these kinds of adaptations "may seek to foreground the oppressive treatment of Ophelia by the men in the play, they finally tend to reiterate the unthreatening child-likeness to which the court in *Hamlet* would like to reduce Ophelia, to which Victorian imagery attempted to confine her" (179).

This chapter's second case study is one of Janet Cardiff's audio walks through Central Park, *Her Long Black Hair* (2004), which Laura Dorwart has described as a work that exemplifies the mad pride movement, and which presents listeners with a "disruptive" and "subversive" representation of Ophelia (4). I depart from Dorwart, however, in arguing that this Ophelia is likewise "frozen" and lacks "the potential for true escape" (12). Whereas Dorwart maintains that Cardiff's walk invites listeners to participate in an imagined community of people who share non-normative ways of thinking, I am more critical of its reliance upon sonic tropes of madness to achieve these ends (13). In this chapter, I compare Mitchell's and Cardiff's adaptations of the *Hamlet* story to identify points of continuity and discontinuity between them and situate them within feminist scholarship. In both case studies, I focus on the two artists' different approaches to staging mad listening, with particular attention to claims around aural intersubjectivity—the ability to listen "with" and "as" another person.

My fourth chapter considers an immersive performance called *Here are the Fragments* (2019), which is based on Frantz Fanon's psychiatric writings on revolutionary listening practices. The playwright, Suvendrini Lena, developed the show over a five-year residency at The Theatre

Centre in Toronto. Notably, Lena is also a neurologist, writer, and professor at the University of Toronto, where she teaches a class called "Staging Medicine." As per the title, *Fragments* mobilizes a combination of sensory experiences including archival materials, whispering voices, live acting, a running narrative, and interviews with people who have the lived experience of voice hearing. Thematically, the show "reflects on the relationships between identity, history, racism, and mental health" and is meant to be experienced ambiently, so as to convey the open-ended experience of mental illness ("No Proscenium"). Echoing familiar rhetoric from my previous case studies, one critic at the *Toronto Star* has called the production "a fascinating simulation of mental illness," and indeed the show features a variety of simulatory devices such as a set of "headphones that echo whoever and whatever is speaking into a microphone at the other end of the room" (Maga para. 6). In this chapter, I attend to the sonic dramaturgies by which Lena simulates mad auralities, particularly in relation to the intersection between anti-Blackness and antimadness.

Building upon the findings of my first four chapters, my fifth takes the form of an autoethnographic study, presented in two forms: a transcript formatted as a series of notes, and an accompanying audio essay. With the support of UBC's Public Scholars Initiative, along with the artistic support of two voice actors and a web designer, this formally inventive chapter is ultimately an experiment in arts-based research—part commentary, part manifesto, part artistic reflection, part lyrical essay, part multimedia piece. Unlike the authorial voice at the heart of my case studies, which maintains a level of critical distance, these notes take a mad first-person standpoint, drawn from my own experience of obsessive–compulsive disorder, depression, and generalized anxiety, among other aspects of my unruly bodymind that evade diagnosis. Challenging the power that diagnoses hold—but not negating their importance for some people—I propose alternative ways of retheorizing these idiosyncratic experiences, through abstract intensities such as "stickiness." By de-medicalizing and depathologizing madness, my goal is to emphasize the persistent ambiguities and slippages of auditory perception that are not so easy to classify. As such, I aim to chart the poetics of the perceptual glitch in relation to mad listening, without the footholds and straightjackets of psychiatric terminology.

Notes

1. For an extensive historical overview of this condition, whose association with insanity goes back much further than the two terms I reference, see Albert Mudry and Robert K. Jackler's "Tracing the Origins of 'Cauliflower Ear' and Its Earlier Names Over Two Millenia" (2020).
2. See William J. Davies's essay, "Autistic Listening" (2019), for another example of a non-essentialized listening which still insists on shared experiences.
3. For research on cultural diversity in sound studies, see *Remapping Sound Studies* (2019), edited by Gavin Steingo and Jim Sykes, who convey the importance of shifting focus toward non-Western sound cultures.
4. For more on the "paranoid" vs. the "reparative" modes in scholarly criticism, see William Cheng's *Just Vibrations: The Purpose of Sounding Good* (2016), which outlines misconceptions on either side.
5. Some of the theoretical frameworks I employ or grapple with include "mad listening" (in my own theorization), "auraldiversity" (John Drever), "acousmatics" (Brian Kane), "forensic aesthetics" (Anna Harpin), "disorientation" (Sara Ahmed), "neuroqueering" (Nick Walker), "mad autoethnography" (Renee Dumaresque), and many others.
6. An earlier description of "close listening" comes from Charles Bernstein, whose 1998 book *Close Listening: Poetry and the Performed Word* argues that spoken poetry is a medium unto itself and that various auditory aspects of poetry—rhythm, prosody, sensuousness—emerge more fully, or resound differently, in oral performance.
7. In *Beyond Immersive Theatre: Aesthetics, Politics and Productive Participation* (2016), Adam Alston defines the experience economy as an "emerging neoliberal paradigm" wherein consumers are "increasingly offered personalised and experiential forms of consumption" (16). Immersive theatre belongs to this paradigm, alongside "theme parks, themed restaurants, experiential marketing, and so on" (16). The concept was first introduced in 1999 by B. Joseph Pine II and James H. Gilmore, in *The Experience Economy: Work Is Theatre & Every Business a Stage*.

8. In his article, "Doing Mad Studies: Making (Non)sense Together" (2016), Richard Ingram glosses the discipline's wider background as follows: "There are many post-Nietzscheans in the twentieth century—Bataille (1954/1988; 1961/1988; 1967/1989), Blanchot (1969/1993; 1973/1992; 1973/1995), Klossowski (1969/1997), Deleuze and Guattari (1972/1983, 1980/1987; Guattari, 1995)—whose work also provides launching points for Mad Studies" (12).
9. See also Therí Alyce Pickens's field-defining literary study, *Black Madness:: Mad Blackness* (2019), which disentangles the conflation of madness and Blackness, and demonstrates the ways that the two experiences operate in tension.
10. To give just one further example, in the course of my research for this book, I alighted upon the nineteenth-century German term "Bühnenwahnsinn," or "stage madness".
11. As Kathryn Church notes in her contribution to *Madness, Distress, and the Politics of Disablement* (2015), "there is a strong tendency for practices to leap the fence. Disabled students march in the Mad Pride Parade; mad-identified students learn how to caption web-docs; deaf/Deaf students provide large-font hand-outs for class presentations; everyone learns to talk in tandem with ASL interpreters (266).
12. In its radical unreasoning, mad studies is enriched by the dream logics of pataphysics. As evidenced by the experimental theory group The Occulture (David Cecchetto, Marc Couroux, Ted Hiebert, Eldritch Priest) this strain of Dadaist philosophy has the potential to move beyond critical analysis and "towards the domain of aesthetics and speculative thought" (Hugill 437). Take, for example, the Earolin, housed in the Musée Patamécanique in Rhode Island—a holographic projection of an ear that plays the violin.
13. For more on visual metaphors of madness, see Ellen Kaplan's "The Cage is My Mind: Object and Image in Depicting Mental Illness on Stage" (2015).

CHAPTER 2

Listening Cures: On Acousmatic Sound in Ridiculusmus's *The Eradication of Schizophrenia in Western Lapland*

Ridiculusmus is a mad-positive theatre company based out of London, England, co-directed by Jon Haynes and David Woods and founded in 1992. Much of the company's repertoire has, in recent years, focused exclusively on mad and disability representation. An important thing to note about the company is that their work reflects personal experience: for an earlier production titled *Yes, Yes, Yes* (1999), they "drew on a lot of mental health experiences, personal and otherwise. It is our light out of depression" ("Yes, Yes, Yes" par. 4). As with other companies, such as Acting Out Productions or May Contain Nuts, whose work focuses on representing lived experience, Ridiculusmus consistently links up with medical professionals to help destigmatize mental health issues. To some extent, however, this sense of medical authority insulates the production from critique, which makes it all the more important to engage critically.

The play at the centre of this chapter is part of a mental health trilogy covering psychosis (*The Eradication of Schizophrenia in Western Lapland*, 2014), post-traumatic stress (*Give Me Your Love*, 2015), and bereavement (*Die! Die! Die! Old People Die!*, 2019). The trilogy, called *Dialogue as the Embodiment of Love,* aims at "a creative interaction between theatre process, mental health therapies and audience experience" (New Adelphi, n.pag). This chapter concerns the first play in the trilogy, *Eradication*, which tells the story of a family—brothers Rupert and Richard, their Mum, Dad, and stepmother Jade (a gynaecologist), a Doctor, and an

M. Tomkinson, *Sound and Sense in Contemporary Theatre*,
https://doi.org/10.1007/978-3-031-78034-9_2

unnamed male patient—all of whom live in the orbit of psychiatric care. After the play's initial run at the Edinburgh Festival, Ridiculusmus was awarded the "Total Theatre Award for Significant Contribution to theatre making in the UK"—which is to say that *Eradication*'s commentary on madness has been widely amplified (Talbot 32). According to one writeup, the play attempts to share "a way of being that remains tantalisingly beyond us" (New Adelphi, n.pag). In the context of this chapter, said "way of being" refers to voice hearing, or so-called "schizophrenia."[1]

This notion of sharing another way of being takes us directly to the central concern of this book: namely, aural simulations of madness. In order, allegedly, to share the auditory symptoms of psychosis with audience members, Ridiculusmus employs a dividing wall that separates the traverse stage, the auditorium, and the auditors into two halves. Consequently, two interlocking scenes are always playing concurrently—one on either side of the wall—and this is meant to create a sense of mock auditory hallucinations. While much of *Eradication*'s promotion and critical response suggests that it provides access to an experience akin to auditory hallucination, I would suggest that this formal analogy operates in a different psychological register than hallucinations, emphasizing something more akin to selective auditory attention. On an affective level, the production's simultaneous scenes and overlapping dialogue encourage disorientation and aural straining. Yet, it is worth applying more pressure to the idea that sonic indeterminacy enables the direct transmission of mad sensory experience to audience members.

To discuss the show's reception in such hyperbolic terms reveals a universalizing impulse. The company, in their own words, wishes to demonstrate that what appears on stage is "not that dissimilar to what you might feel on a daily basis" (17). This line of thinking suggests that there is some perceptual glitch in all of us that draws comparison to psychosis, and that the production in question aims to highlight this supposedly inherent quality to promote empathy. Lacking in the discourse around this play, however, is a clear delineation of analogy and lived experience when it comes to voice hearing.

In this chapter, I will consider how Haynes and Woods stage madness through sound. Before getting to a close analysis of the play, I begin with a discussion of the problematics of disability simulation, which grounds this and all subsequent chapters. What, I ask, are some of the ethical problems with imagining that this production's stage design, novel as it is, approximates the lived experience of voice hearing, and what phenomenological problems arise from treating soundscapes as mindscapes? Moreover, what are the ethical contours of such attempts to simulate madness through sound? Strikingly, through my analysis of the play's critical reception, I found many interlocutors who both describe madness simulation in absolute terms while simultaneously championing the play's ambiguities.[2] Navigating a middle path between these paradoxical impulses, I focus on detailing and unpacking the company's representational strategies.

To that end, this chapter scrutinizes the play's dividing wall as a sound object, asking how it mediates madness and becomes instrumentalized in mad listening. I contend that sonic intersubjectivity is always a function of what philosopher François J. Bonnet calls desiring-listening, which refers to the way that "listening fictionalizes the relation to the audible" (140). One major function of the play's dividing wall, like the veil behind which Pythagoras was said to lecture, is to sustain this fiction. As sound studies scholar Brian Kane suggests, acousmatic sound "is often deployed in order to grant auditory access to transcendental spheres, different in kind from the purely sonic effect—a way of listening to essence, truth, profundity, ineffability, or interiority" (9). Acousmatic sound—i.e., any sound whose source is obscured, not necessarily in relation to vision—thus makes way for transcendental claims about simulating the listening positionality of the mad subject (falsely imagined as being singular). Kane reminds us of the pathological context of the term in the late nineteenth century, when the term "acousmatic" was synonymous with hallucination and referred to "a species of depraved hearing in which sounds are imagined as if they were really heard" (92). Throughout the period, according to Kane, there are frequent associations of acousmatic sounds with horror and the uncanny, strange noises emanating from crypts and castles (92).

In relation to *Eradication*, the transcendent might be thought of as unmediated access to the auditory experience of the other. Versions of this claim emerge from multiple sources, including the company itself, as well as discourse surrounding the production, and previous scholarly commentary. Writing against this transcendent strain of thought, I submit that there are hard limits to intersubjective listening, that listening-as-other functions largely within the realm of analogy, and that the more theoretically sound approach to simulated madness is not to perpetuate this fantasy in the name of decreasing stigma and increasing empathy, but rather to attend in detail to the formal operations governing such analogies. At stake here is the difference between lived experience and material metaphor, mad phenomenology, and mad phenomenal analogy. Ridiculusmus's play harbours these tensions but does not exactly come down on either side as a matter of principle. As such, it is a valuable case study in the problems of what might be called *normalization through democratization*. "The idea of democratization," says Anja Drautzburg, "relates to the fact that everyone present in the auditorium hears voices and that, ultimately, audiences are encouraged to call into question categorizations such as 'sane' and 'mad'" (174). I concur with the author's observation that audiences are led to question these categories; however, the gesture towards democratization relies on audist assumptions about everyone hearing to the same degree and in the exact same way. The problem with the democratization theory is that it turns hearing madly into a matter of fact, as though the production simply produces an effect (i.e., the auditory hallucination) which is then neatly received by the audience. It also elides perceptual differences, most explicitly those of deaf and hard-of-hearing audience members. Just as the company "didn't want it to be obvious who was the mad person in the play," according to Haynes, so too is the difference elided between lived madness and stage madness (Talbot 17).

Listening Context

Writing, as I am, in the midst of a global pandemic, my experience of the play was more heavily mediated than might be expected for a typical case study. I watched the performance on the company's Vimeo page, with a link graciously provided by the directors. I must admit, then, that I am at multiple layers of remove in theorizing the wall, the acoustic properties of the room, and the audience's reception. The wall, as such, lives behind yet another wall—my computer screen—and every echo of the performance space comes to me through a set of over-ear headphones. Format-wise, Ridiculusmus has opted for a split-screen video to offer something resembling the live experience, but repeated viewings in this mode offer a much finer interpretive grain that I would have had in person—not least of all because I am able to see both sides of the stage at once in the video, and the volume has been equalized so that I can also hear both sides of the split stage with the same amount of clarity. As such, the video clearly tidies up aspects of the performance that would otherwise be more ambiguous, and quite literally takes what was most opaque about the live show and makes it transparent. Nonetheless, I would suggest that these intermedial differences do not pose a significant problem to my analysis, since my focus is not on evaluating how well the play's madness simulations work. To suggest that the video fails in some way to capture the effect of the mock-hallucinations in a live context is to miss the point, since I am troubling the notion of simulation altogether.

Thus far, theatre scholars such as Anja Drautzburg, James Frieze, Nicola Shaughnessy, and Jon Venn have been in agreement in suggesting that this play's representation of madness is politically productive, citing its use of polyvocality, dialogism, strategic ambiguity, and tolerance of uncertainty. In the analysis that follows, I aim to complicate this view by showing that the discourse surrounding this play is less tolerant of uncertainty than it might seem. A narrow focus on the play's representations of mad aurality will help us challenge certain unspoken and unchallenged assumptions about *Eradication*'s sonic politics.

Theatrical Context and Theoretical Background

Though the play is not immersive in the interactive sense, it is nonetheless informed by immersive techniques. Indeed, Talbot positions the play within a "wider context of theatrical experiments with audience immersion and agency" (8). Haynes and Woods have also said that, from the outset, they didn't want to make "a straight, kind of normal theatre show" (8). When the work premiered in 2014, the online immersive theatre database, *No Proscenium*, had just been formed, and well-known critics such as Lyn Gardner were just starting to pose lofty questions about this still-emerging genre: "Should immersive theatre audiences accept greater responsibility?" and "Should we follow the instructions written by the artist, or should we refuse and thereby create an outcome different to the one that ensues when the instructions are followed?" (n.pag).[3] Along similar lines, Adam Alston has described a variety of immersive theatre productions as "affective texts" that are co-created with audience members, who are presented with a kind of social script for sensory engagement. Audiences of the play in question might agree to suspend their disbelief around madness simulations, for example, not unlike a stagehand might agree to look surprised when sawn in half.

Premiering in the middle of an immersion boom, *Eradication* took influence from big-name theatre companies such as Shunt, based in London, who were producing immersive work in the early 2000s, before the term was popularized. Other formal inspiration came not from theatre but from an experimental psychiatric treatment called "Open Dialogue" (OD). This is a community-based treatment method for psychosis created, as the play's title tells us, in Western Lapland. The treatment entails "generating a therapeutic process that can tolerate uncertainty in order to mobilize the psychological resources of the family and the social network" (Seikkula et al. 194). The clinical psychologist Anne Cooke, in her review of the play, says that the aim of this methodology is to foster a dialogue in which everyone's voice is heard and respected. No one person's view of the situation is privileged, including the clinician's. The emphasis is on "being with," rather than "doing to" (422). According to Jon Venn, who writes about madness representations in contemporary British theatre, this alternative form of treatment is also inspired by philosopher Mikael Bakhtin's notion of dialogism, which suggests that the formation of meaning is inherently relational, and thus we find the patient in OD therapy situated within a network of perspectives and a "cacophony of voices" (98). Venn argues that, while the play is not directly modelled after an OD session, it nonetheless "allows the audience to undergo a psychological revelation, a therapeutic process, a curing" (99).

An Overview of the Play

Written by David Woods and Jon Haynes, *Eradication* follows two brothers, Rupert and Richard, along with their Mum, Dad, stepmother Jade (a gynaecologist), a Doctor, and an unnamed male patient (note: the Dad and Jade characters are ventriloquized by the Doctor and Mum, and never actually appear in the flesh). The original cast included—and the cast in my reference video includes—David Woods (Doctor), Jon Haynes (Richard), Patrizia Paolini (Mum), and Richard Talbot (Rupert).

Because *Eradication* involves a complex interleaving of scenes, it is difficult to summarize linearly. Across different reviews and critiques of the play, one will find descriptions of various scenes that are absent in this filmed version and were only added later. Since tracking these changes will not be much use to the present analysis, I will focus exclusively on relating the version of the play that I saw, filmed in March of 2014 in London at Shoreditch Town Hall, a multipurpose community space not necessarily designed with acoustics in mind.

And because so many differences exist between the playtext, the filmed performance, and subsequent performances, indexing these changes exhaustively would make for a chapter unto itself. Suffice it to say that the two most significant differences in the film version include the presence of a spoken chorus in between the acts, and the absence of a standalone second act, "Betty." In this early version of the play, about a quarter of the second act, as written in the playtext, is nested within the third act. Frieze describes the second act (as written) as "a scene in which the brothers interact with their father and his new wife, Jade, on the day of the wedding" (182). The filmed version, however, makes no mention of the wedding, focusing instead on a doll named "Betty" that Richard blames his stepmother, Jade, for throwing away.

The play's first act, "Chaos," and the third act, "Clarity," are staged simultaneously, though the former is set five to ten years in the past. Recall that the venue's traverse stage is divided into two halves, with two interweaving narratives and interlocking dialogue, and two audiences—one on either side. Each half of the play is set in a different time period: one side of the stage shows a domestic scene, which is the first act, "Chaos," and which Ridiculusmus has variably called the "family side" or the "domestic side" or the "private side" (Talbot 9). Meanwhile, the third act, "Clarity," is staged on the "public" side, where the stage depicts a doctor's consulting room (9).

As a whole, the play depicts a family in crisis, with Mum's experience of madness set in the past on the private side and her son Richard's experience of madness set in the future on the public side. Richard has had a breakdown and is in a psychiatric hospital, where he is being treated by a Doctor. Mum is at home with Rupert, her other son who looks after her and spends a lot of time on his phone. The two of them are waiting for Dad to come home and talking mostly about food. Conversations on the private side tend towards the quotidian, while topics on the public side gravitate towards psychiatry and fantasy. The Doctor and Richard both wander between the two halves of the stage through a centre door, further linking the already-linked stories together. Occasionally, there is a back-and-forth between the two sides of the stage where dialogue becomes triangulated. At one point, for example, Mum tells Rupert that "Dracula was from Ireland" while Richard, on the other side of the stage, tells the Doctor that he has a "spectacularly large" mind; and then Rupert, responding to both of these assertions at once, says "bollocks" (*Eradication* 00:03:30–00:04:16).

It is in precisely this fashion that Ridiculusmus attempts to stage polyphony and family dialogue, modelled on Open Dialogue and its principle of tolerating uncertainty. The question becomes: who was Rupert responding to, Richard or Mum? This effect also characterizes the hallucinatory quality that the audience on the public side is meant to experience, in that the word "bollocks" seems to emanate from within Richard's mind, as though a second voice within himself was responding to him internally. Some moments of interlocking dialogue are less discernible, however. In certain moments, the dialogue fully overlaps and becomes difficult to parse, even with the forensic capabilities afforded by video playback. In this manner, the dialogue moves constantly between synchronicity, asynchronicity, and disharmony.

Though the play is hardly linear, and its polyphony is not reducible to paragraph-form, it might be useful to have a sense of the general plot before moving forward: at the top of the show, we encounter a chorus (as I mentioned above, this is cut in later versions), who describe two feuding brothers, before opening on a silent stage, where Mum stands beside Rupert, who plays with his phone while the Doctor sits alone on the other side of the wall. Mum says that she has made fish pie while Richard approaches with a large knife in hand. Richard then crosses through the stage's centre door and hands this knife to the Doctor, who holds it while seeming to eavesdrop from the other side. Richard introduces himself to the private side as a writer, before crossing over onto the public side—the future—where he is now in therapy. On the public side, Richard describes himself in grandiose terms, suggesting that he is the true author of various canonical works of fiction, which he claims to have written under different aliases including Vladimir Nabokov and Edna O'Brien. On the private side, Rupert pesters his Mum about what's for dinner. Then, Richard crosses back over and the Doctor quotes R.D. Laing at length, describing the impossibility of experiencing other's experiences. Around this point, Mum hears a voice (which is implied to be the Doctor's) and asks who it is. She goes to the wall and tries to look and hear beyond it, peeling back the curtain. Mum tells Richard that she is in treatment for an unnamed condition. Mum talks about how Dracula is actually from Ireland while Richard, on the other side of the wall, talks about his Mum in the past tense, telling the Doctor that she lost her mind. The Doctor then moves to the wall and tries to spy and eavesdrop across the barrier. Richard then crosses back to the private side and tells Mum that he has a girlfriend who is trans, while Rupert swaps sides with him and shakes a pill bottle in a series of awkward jerks. Swapping sides again, Rupert tells Mum that the house is haunted, while the Doctor, comparing Richard's mind to a house, tells him that trauma is a hole in the roof that needs patching (there are many such moments of thematic overlap in the play). The Doctor tells Richard about a talk-therapy treatment that has eradicated schizophrenia in Western Lapland without the use of prescription drugs. Rupert asks Mum what's for dinner, and the Doctor responds "Pardon?" from his side of the wall, implying that he too is prone to hallucinatory mishearings. Because his job is on the line and he cannot pursue the Lapland treatment, The Doctor prescribes drugs to Richard, who then takes these pills to the other side of the stage and gives them to Mum, who refuses to take them. At this point, the Doctor makes an angry phone call about signing divorce papers. Mum and Rupert talk about what's for dinner while Richard, returning to the public side, talks to the Doctor about hearing voices. Richard tells the Doctor he watched a documentary and when the Doctor asks what it was about he replies "gorillas" while his Mum says "fish fingers" in quick succession (*Eradication* 00:29:16–00:29:19). Richard then relates a story to the doctor about a time he saw his mother in Russell Square, acting like a frog. Here, Mum begins to croak on the other side of the stage. Becoming more agitated, Mum hops around like a frog and then rips the curtains off the wall, revealing both audiences to each other. Suddenly, the characters start folk dancing to a Finnish tune, sashaying freely from one side of the stage to the other, linking arms and leapfrogging over each other's backs. This marks the end of the first and third acts, after which there is an intermission and the audience changes sides to see what they previously heard and vice versa. After one full repetition, including the nested second act I mentioned above, the play ends once again on the torn-down curtain, with both audiences revealed to each other. The playtext, however, has the narrative conclude with Rupert being hit by a car and the characters "returning with head in bloodied hands" (93). Drautzburg describes this ending as "an accident to explain the trauma experienced by the family," but notes that Ridiculusmus had dropped this ending by the time of the Shoreditch performance (178).

Notably, the company's representations of madness and psychiatry have changed significantly since their earliest work, wherein they "were embracing almost stereotypical representations of madness" (*Performing Psychologies* 17). In an interview with Richard Talbot, who played Rupert and was a creative collaborator in this production, Haynes and Woods "claim to have rejected both 'mad acting' and acting 'mad,'" which perhaps raises certain questions about the paradoxes of playing mad characters without acting mad (1). To reject mad acting in a play about madness, in other words, might mean a missed opportunity to interrogate one's own representational strategies. Another quote from this interview that potentially undercuts mad-positive representations is Haynes's comment suggesting that "if you put madness on the stage you wouldn't want to look at it. It's actually really horrible" (17). Such statements highlight an awkward contradiction at the core of *Eradication*'s dramaturgy. By one measure, the company wants to preserve a sense of ambiguity with regards to who is mad and who is sane on stage. But by another, it is implied that a truly mad character would be too easy to identify. The former implies that we are all mad in some way, while the latter implies that madness is fully other.

Even still, the question remains as to whether it is possible to listen across subjectivities. Even if everyone in an audience identifies as mad, is everyone's "delirium" not different in degree and kind? The preoccupation with transmitting, sharing, and simulating perception is endemic to contemporary theatre, especially theatres of madness and disability, where there is often an explicit emphasis on audience identification and empathy. Accordingly, as a work of sound and mad studies, this chapter aims to assess this preoccupation with reference to an array of critical terms that I develop here: mad phenomenal analogy, mad aural mimesis, and mad point of audition. Following an overview of the latter concept, which helps contextualize my approach, I move towards a close analysis of the performance and its reception.

Mad Point of Audition

The term "point of audition" comes from film studies, where it refers to the aural equivalent of the point of view shot. The most recognizable instances of this technique include when shells go off in war movies and the character's ears ring, or when someone puts on headphones in a movie and the external sound world disappears. Film studies scholar Rick Altman says that "this technique locates us in a very specific place—the body of the character who hears for us" (61). Altman tells us that point of audition sound "constitutes the perfect interpellation" because it invites us to "identify with someone who will hear for us" (60). In some cases, point of audition sound is used to approximate another person's psychological subject position. According to Michel Chion, who coined the term, point of audition sound not only positions us within the "subjective designation" of the character through whom we hear, but also situates us within mediatized space, hearing from certain angles and auditory vantage points (89). Keeping in mind audist assumptions, however, we should take "hearing" to mean something far more capacious than what is implied by normative audition.

Mindful of this problem, I argue that the point of audition, as a representational tactic, also applies to the theatre, though it has rarely, if ever, been discussed in this context. It is fairly uncontroversial, however, to suggest that sound effects on the stage can still have the effect of positioning audience members subjectively and spatially. The play in question, *Eradication*, is a case in point, since it attempts to position audience members in the headspace of its characters via the aforementioned dividing wall.

With regards to its construction of a mad point of audition, much theorizing around *Eradication* has been conducted in an appreciative mode, taking for granted that the play's goal of simulating hallucinations has been effective and that the success of said simulation engenders a feeling of greater empathy towards mad people. If simulations have been designed to encourage intersubjectivity and empathy through placing the spectator or auditor in another's metaphorical shoes, then point of audition sound approximates a kind of intangible shoe for one's ear. Though not in use here, headphones make this effect all the more tangible, which is evident from the fact that binaural recording devices are sometimes called Head and Torso Simulators (HATS). These devices aim to recreate the acoustic properties of a universal human body (in actuality: a mannequin) and how sound would enter that body's ears and resonate therein. These heads also model an "average" head-related transfer function (HRTF), which refers to the way that one's individual physiology interacts with the acoustical properties of incoming sounds and alters those sounds accordingly. Here, the terminology and technology itself begins to explain how point of audition sound might be constructed—not just through reverberation or equalization, but through altering the shape of the recording tools.

The play in question, however, relies almost exclusively on live sound. Its mediating technology, as I have suggested, is the dividing wall. The wall, as an acousmatic screen, provides the material means of simulation. More than materially altering the sounds that it interacts with, the wall gives a psychic structure to these sounds. Just as a character in a film might jump into a swimming pool and the soundscape would suddenly become dull and bubbly, the audience member at this production is meant to listen *through* the wall (as through the water). The wall, as a sound object, is thus a mediating substance of sorts. It intervenes in one's listening, reshaping it to conform to an allegedly mad point of audition. It proclaims that hearing voices within a state of psychosis is similar, in some way, to hearing voices through a wall. It implies that to hear madly is to hear dully, distantly, differently, distractedly, dauntingly, discordantly, and disorientedly—among other metaphors. In this regard, the wall functions as both a visual, sonic, and material metaphor: as Anna Harpin puts it, such material entities have the potential to "disturb notions and associations of space, place, and perception" *(Performance* 194). To illustrate her argument, Harpin cites Caryl Churchill's innovative play concerning postpartum psychosis and possession, *The Skriker* (1994), and argues that its extravagant wordplay conspires "to create an ethical translation of the presumed unintelligibility of psychosis into meaningful theatrical communication" (203). Arguably, the logics, aesthetics, and significations of the dividing wall offer a comparable material means to trouble, translate, and communicate experiences of voice hearing theatrically. In other words, the wall structures the experience of voice hearing into a series of "surface expressions" for theatrical engagement (206).

Of course, the listener also actively participates in this meaning-making. According to sound artist and scholar Lawrence English: "The listener becomes a performer in place, amplifying and refocusing temporal and spatial phenomena not merely through physiological means, but also via active theoretical and methodological frameworks" (2). Though Haynes and Woods have allegedly rejected mad acting, perhaps what they have really done is displace this responsibility onto the auditor. In some sense, the audience members of this play are the ones who are performing madness through the theoretical framework of simulation. Though Ridiculusmus does not advance an explicit framework of theatrical simulation, this term perhaps comes closest to describing the conditions of reception in which there is an attempt to reproduce a perceptual event. Indeed, Scott Magelssen has suggested that simulations can also be thought of as "likenesses," and share the linguistic connotations of the simile, insofar as simulations are "meant to strike a comparison" (9).

Eradication's madness simulation requires audience members to suspend their disbelief and participate, imaginatively, in the fantasy of intersubjectivity. Advancing a theory of relational listening, and drawing upon philosopher Peter Szendy, Lawrence asks the same question I have been asking throughout this chapter so far: "Can one make a listening listened to? Can I transmit my listening, unique as it is?" (4). Though not responding directly to Szendy, sound studies scholar Jonathan Sterne strongly denies this possibility when he says: "People have no direct intellectual or experiential access to the faculty of hearing in its supposed state of nature. We can posit that the interiority of experience exists and try to describe it, but that access is always mediated. We can't even hear ourselves hearing, or not hearing" (72). To quote Sterne at greater length, since he puts it so well:

> What would sound studies become if we began without the automatic assumptions that we have direct, full access to our own hearing, or through our hearing, direct access to the sonic world, or through the sonic world, intersubjectivity with others? Such a project is a little difficult to imagine, but it would at least substitute a new set of problems for the ones that come from idealizing hearing and idealizing ourselves as perfect auditors. If no sound is possible without hearing, then sound studies – but also many forms of polities – begins with hearing the hearing of others. (74)

With this provocation to the discipline in mind, the remainder of this chapter is dedicated to exploring the mad point of audition in more depth, bringing together the concepts discussed so far in a close analysis of the performance. My writing is particularly invested in interpreting the function of the wall within the "signal chain of audition" and asking how it operates within the play's simulation of madness (Feaster 142). To what extent, I wonder, does the wall ostensibly stand in for a mad person's psychophysiology as a kind of abstract variation on the head simulator?

Close Listening

What's lacking in scholarship around this play, and what's also lacking in the intersecting fields of mad studies and sound studies, is a theory—or an assemblage of theories—about mad listening. In her writing about aurality, Lynne Kendrick asks a question that we might pose to *Eradication* as we move towards developing such a theory: "How does the sonorous world invite experience, sensation and immersion?" (xxiv). Kendrick's notion of an invitation allows for a certain amount of open-endedness that is often missing when we say that a work of art conclusively achieves the things it sets out to do. Because studying aurality is about finding a balance between production, reception, and everything that happens in between, we ought to weigh the discursive and phenomenological fields of reception against the legislative conditions of production. Take the following quote from one of the play's directors, Woods, for example: "We've got this incredibly complex script that gives you the experience of auditory hallucination, as best we can; it's a sort of chaotic immersion into the experience of psychoses, which is quite unpleasant and difficult to deal with" ("Inside" 05:30–05:55). These are the play's legislative conditions of listening: complexity, hallucination, immersion, psychosis, unpleasantness and difficulty. But not everyone will experience these things in the same way. Moreover, doing the "best one can" to approximate the experience of auditory hallucinations only further validates the applicability of terms like "simulation" and "metaphor" to describe the production's technical aims.

According to one critic, *Eradication* "challenges how you listen and fathom what you hear" (Costa). According to another, the play is "aurally remarkable, as the plays alternate between interrupting, obstructing, and echoing each other (Brennan)." When critics use descriptors such as "challenging" and "remarkable" to describe the play's unique staging and soundscape, we are in the realm of the discursive. These concepts structure one's listening, insofar as this language primes an audience for certain modes of engagement. What makes some sounds challenging and others remarkable? Your answer will be different from mine. Yet another critic of the play says that it is "unsettling to hear a muffled show that we cannot see" (Bano). We might narrow in on the "muffled" as a specific typology of sound in *Eradication*, understood as a subcategory of noise in Kendrick's sense of those sounds which exceed understanding (104). The muffled sound lies beyond the senses but also exceeds sense. Its timbral quality suggests a lack of high-end clarity, and therefore a lack of information. Muffledness is associated with hearing loss and the ear itself, but it can also be a spatial, acoustical, and architectural condition, as in the case of the play's dividing wall. With muffledness, a degree of separation and alienation is implied. The partial occultation of sounds beyond the wall is, as I discussed above, one of the central features of acousmatic listening. "Acousmatic sounds," according to Kane, "encourage the imaginative projection of a sonic body" (8) and this body "is taken to be transcendent" (9). An acousmatic trope of sorts, muffledness in this play carries an association with madness, with voice hearing, and with a transcendent sonic body—namely: that of the actors on the far side of the wall, who Woods and Haynes conceptualize as quasi-hallucinatory. In *Eradication*, muffledness is a form of sonic underdetermination that simultaneously resists and encourages close listening.

Madness and Sound Design

In this section, I offer a close listening of two of the play's most noteworthy sound effects: a rattling pill bottle and a croaking frog noise. By listening closely to the play's sound design, I aim to show how each of these effects operates as a metaphor for madness within the framework of mad aurality. Throughout this discussion, I relate these metaphors back to my primary concerns with madness simulation, intersubjectivity, and empathy. One scene in particular emphasizes the interplay between the critical tensions I have noted so far. Monologuing at length from one of R.D. Laing's anti-psychiatric texts, the play's Doctor character says:

> My experience of you is not inside me. It is simply you as I experience you. And I do not experience you as inside me. Similarly you do not experience me as inside you. [...] My experience of you is just another form of words for 'you as I experience you' and 'your experience of me' equals 'me as you experience me'. [...] Your experience of me is not inside you. [...] My experience of you is invisible to you. [...] I cannot experience your experience. [...] You cannot experience my experience. [...]. (*Eradication* 51–52)

Here, in a metatheatrical fashion, the Doctor acknowledges the potential shortcomings of, and paradoxes within, the play's attempt to reproduce auditory hallucinations. As Anja Drautzburg says about this scene, the Doctor "might be telling the spectators that it is impossible to empathise with the mad characters on stage if they have not experienced mental distress themselves" (175). Drautzburg proposes that this self-referential Laingian critique has a metacognitive effect, whereby audience members are made to question their own perceptual frames (176). However, she then goes on to say that in such moments, an audience member's "own lived experience of madness" unites with the "reality of mental distress

[...] that the play evokes" (178). In her analysis of the play, Drautzburg advances Christopher Dingwall-Jones's theory of radical empathy, which is itself borrowed from Matthew Ratcliffe's phenomenological study of empathy. Dingwall-Jones suggests that there can be no straightforward insight into another's experience, but that both subjects' experiences can be transposed, "creating a space of shared subjectivity" (48). For him, the moment of the "break" is most important, wherein a person recognizes the limitations of their understanding (51). Dingwall-Jones says that the moment of recognition—the break—ultimately "disrupts the impression that these performances are a totalizing attempt to represent 'what mental illness is like'" (59). Performances that emphasize this break, he continues, "shy away from claims to representational truth in favour of capturing something of an affective experience" (59). This strategy, he concludes, is "properly ethical" (59). However, what I have been suggesting throughout this chapter is that *Eradication* offers a mixed message when it comes to claims of representational fidelity.

Whereas Dingwall-Jones's argument advances the kind of nuance I have been looking for, I have noted a tendency elsewhere for critics and scholars to discuss the play at large in terms of productive ambiguity while discussing auditory hallucinations in suspiciously absolute terms. Drautzburg, for example, suggests that "the split stage and the simultaneity are the technical vehicles for recreating the effect of auditory hallucinations. In fact, the audience actually experiences auditory hallucinations in the sense that the spectators hear voices but cannot control, identify, or make sense of them" (165). Note how the metaphoricity of madness simulation has been tuned out in this example. Moreover, there is no matter of degree or spectrum applied to these claims. Can the audience not make partial sense of these sounds, and can they not exercise some amount of control in identifying and assigning them? There is an implicit thesis about mad listening here that groups together auditory hallucinations with, say, global aphasia. The implication is that mad listening is not just epistemically messy but totally disordered and completely devoid of reason. This, I would argue, is one of the key issues with trying to simulate madness through sound: there is an overeagerness to draw spurious connections between formal strategies such as polyphony and perceptual experiences such as voice hearing.[4] An audience member might identify a voice on the other side of the play's dividing wall through a simple act of deduction, having flipped through a playbill before the performance. People with the lived experience of voice hearing might not necessarily have such contextual footholds. This is just one of many potential gaps between simulated madness and the lived experience of madness, including Sterne's crucial point that such representations are almost always too stable, failing to account for the discontinuities of disability over time (14).

As I mentioned at the outset of this chapter, Ridiculusmus uses strategic ambiguity in the form of dialogism and polyphony, often towards anxiogenic ends. Writing about the overwhelm of epistemic noise, philosopher of technology Cecile Malaspina suggests that the "mental state of noise" can be attributed to information overload (93). Doubtless, overload is one of the consequences of polyphony. Though Ridiculusmus does not advance a psychiatric theory of noise, such a theory is implicit in their attempt to convey the experience of auditory hallucinations. I would suggest that one of these unnamed strategies revolves around sensory gating or the cocktail party effect, in which audiences are bombarded with auditory stimuli in the form of simultaneous conversations. To reproduce the sensation of increased auditory stimuli associated with hallucinations, the directors use overlapping dialogue to frustrate the audience's ability to separate meaningful and non-meaningful information. Watching and listening to the play is an exercise in selective attention. The word "attention" is a bat signal of sorts for theatre and sound studies scholar George Home-Cook, who asks an important question for our purposes: "how does theatre 'construct' and present 'objects' for the attention of its audience and what happens when we begin to describe how these intended percepts are manifestly perceived and articulated by means of theatrical attention?" (42). Since attention deficits are commonly described in a wide variety of diagnoses, I would suggest that this fact alone complicates the relevance of a voice hearing simulation based solely on polyphony. To hear many voices at once, and to have trouble distinguishing them, is as much a feature of going to the pub on a Saturday night as it is a feature of attending the play in question, though our expectations of these two sonic environments may differ dramatically. This is just one contradiction at the centre of *Eradication*'s experiment in madness simulation: if auditory hallucination is normalized as a fact of everyday life for everyone everywhere, then why do we require extra devices such as the dividing wall to create an immersive context for mad listening? Moreover, if the cocktail party effect applies to a majority of neurotypical people, then what is mad about this form of listening? If this effect fails to apply to deaf or hard-of-hearing people, then what is universal about this mode of listening? And if this effect carries pathological associations with other diagnoses, then what is specific to auditory hallucination in this mode of listening? Finally, if the experience of auditory hallucination is one that's shared or shareable by all, then why is the play explicitly concerned with curing and "eradicating" so-called schizophrenia?

Staying on the subject of curative logic, and returning to Home-Cook's question about objects of attention, I want to focus on one of the play's most curious sound objects: the pill bottle. We first hear this prop when Rupert passes from the private to the public side of the stage, greeting the Doctor, who rattles a bottle of pills five times in a Pavlovian come-and-get-them gesture, without actually saying as much, before handing the bottle to his patient. Rupert then enters into a jittery dance with the bottle in hand, clicking the safety seal, shaking the bottle in random, almost musical bursts. As if it has a will of its own, the bottle also seems to shake him, as though it is a Pandora's box containing something restless that wants to escape. The stage directions simply read "Doctor administers drugs," but the performative act of administration is rendered highly abstract and choreographic (27). More than choreographic, this act is also transformed into a sound event. More specifically, the sound of the pill bottle is both an event and an object; it is a sound event in the composer R. Murray Schafer's sense of a sound considered within a "situated spatial and cultural context" but it is also a sound object in composer Pierre Schaeffer's sense of a sound removed from its original context of signification (Kane 151). According to Kane, Shafer's sound event is associated with known causes and sources. This means knowing with absolute certainty that the object being shaken is a pill bottle because its sonic fingerprint is completely unique. A sound object, by contrast, is supposedly "ontologically distinct from its source," a medium unto itself (156).

The rattling of the pill bottle is an index that points towards medication being administered. But in establishing an acousmatic situation, the dividing wall casts doubt on the indexicality of the rattling.[5] Perhaps someone might hear a rain stick, a box of jewelery, a jar of beans, a caxixi, a loudspeaker, or nothing at all. As Kane puts it: "Sound is always in danger of being apprehended as something other than itself" (25). It is clear that Woods and Haynes deliberately play with such misapprehensions. In the actor's hands, the pill bottle makes a shift towards non-indexicality the moment he starts shaking it like a musical instrument.

Prompting a shift in attention away from indexical listening (Schaeffer's *écouter*), Woods and Haynes abstract the pill bottle by playing with its signifying power, turning it into a sound object such that the audience might focus more on the bottle's essential percussive qualities than its identity (non-indexical listening or *entendre*). As a sound object, the pill bottle becomes immaterial and non-signifying, reduced to its autonomous effects: a high-pitched rattling of plastic and particulate.

Once again, the question of intersubjectivity rears its head—that is: does every hearing audience member perceive the same object? "Under what conditions can an object be identified?" asks Kane (19). Citing the phenomenologist Edmund Husserl, Kane suggests that the listening subject synthesizes a unified sound from their own set of associations, be they cultural, psychological, contextual, and so on (21). For Schaeffer, "the transcendence of the object is shared by multiple subjects, thus presupposing a shared objective world" (22). Applied to the present analysis, this would suggest that everyone in the audience hears a pill bottle—end of story. However, the problem with any theory of intersubjective agreement between listeners is that it assumes a normative audience. In this regard, *Eradication* cannot have its cake of madness simulation and eat it too vis-à-vis intersubjective empathy. I take the position, contra Schaeffer, that there can be no pure sound object: the sound of the pill bottle will always have "worldly affiliations," to use Kane's term (148). For Kane, the acousmatic listening situation is defined by an irresolvable anxious tension that neither reduces sounds to their causes nor separates them completely. But note how this tension is ultimately dissolved when the audience swaps sides between the acts. Assuming a normative spectator-auditor, those who previously heard the pill bottle can now see it and hear it for a second time. This disclosure of the sound source breaks the illusion, stripping the pill bottle of its acousmaticity (one's perception of a sound as being acousmatic) in the moment of de- or dis-acousmatization (the moment the sound source is ascertained).

What should we make of this gesture towards perceptual security? If tolerance of uncertainty is one of Ridiculusmus's key aesthetic values in this play, then why reveal the true source of the sound? As Talbot puts it: "After the interval some audience members experience more clarity because what appeared distant and inaccessible is now visible and clearly audible" (6). To what extent does this move towards clarification square with the company's attempt to simulate auditory hallucinations as best they can? Whose lived experience of psychosis or voice hearing is accurately represented by this moment of sudden theatrical relief? I would argue that the company's drive to reduce the pill bottle to its banal causes—a "drive to dis-acousmatize sound," in Kane's terms—further disconnects the play from mad phenomenology (156). The audience's uncertainties and anxieties are dispelled on both a cognitive and affective level, respectively. Implicitly, then, there exists a fundamental tension between dramaturgical closure and mad phenomenology. A more productive and faithful form of mad listening, in my estimation, would mean allowing for acousmatic uncertainty to linger. One imagines the uncanny possibilities of a pill bottle that looks and sounds subtly different the second time it is shaken, such that the bottle's second audience wouldn't know whether this was a confirmation of their previous hypothesis or another layer of uncertainty. And so it is with all of the sounds that are made familiar as a result of the audience's repositioning: how can uncertainty be better tolerated?

Though anxiety-based simulations can inadvertently worsen stigma, there is an altogether different sort of anxiety at the heart of acousmatic listening that has less to do with pathologization and more to do with perceptual disorientation. It might help us to think of acousmatic listening and mad listening (or, at least, simulations of mad listening) as two totally distinct modes. My argument is that what Ridiculusmus considers to be a madness simulation is actually an acousmatic listening situation framed in the wrong terms. The problem, from the outset, lies in framing the play in terms of approximating hallucinations rather than acousmatics. By framing the play in these terms, the audience's anxieties are projected onto people who experience auditory hallucinations. Following Bree Hadley, I note that when artists "equip spectators with ready-made readings and responses" it serves to protect them "from truly having to truly encounter the other, or take responsibility for their relation to the other, in the street or on the stage" (7). If Ridiculusmus were to remove the play's simulatory framework—perhaps by discussing the listening situation exclusively in terms of acousmatics—then the resulting anxieties might be understood in less freighted terms and received with fewer stigmatic associations. If sonic empathy is the intended outcome of such simulations, what type of knowledge of the voice hearing experience does the audience come away with here? A gentle corrective, here, might be to insist ever more on the play's fictional listening situation than its fidelity to mad sensory experience.

Tuning into another sound effect now, the remainder of this chapter considers the ways in which the aforementioned themes intersect with gendered aspects of mad sound and mad listening within the play. The sound effect in question is that of a frog, as impersonated by the Mum character. Writing about the gendering of sound, Anne Carson reminds us that "madness and witchery as well as bestiality are conditions commonly associated with the use of the female voice in public, in ancient as well as modern contexts" (2). Troubling such associations, Carson asks an important question: "How do our presumptions about gender affect the way we hear sounds?" (11). Because Ridiculusmus frame madness in a semi-spectacularized way, with elements of clowning, it is not always easy to tell what is being presumed and what is being played with. The company tends to double down on aesthetic norms for the sake of recontextualizing them. Early in the play, for example, Richard is shown carrying a carving knife, an image Woods and Haynes deploy as an explicit statement: "That carving knife in the show was to say, 'We acknowledge that carving knives are associated with madness.' But we wanted to subvert that" (Talbot 26). Transferring this logic to the play's representation of gendered madness, one notes that Richard's mother is represented in a similarly absurdist fashion. As the play's only female character, she comes to embody a frog, croaking and hopping around on all fours around the stage, before rising to her feet, wrapping herself up in the dividing wall's curtains, ripping them off to expose the other side of the stage, all the while repeatedly shouting "I can't stop" (*Eradication* 00:30:50–00:31:05). Despite this scene's murky ironies, it is difficult not to interpret this scene through the critical lens of reinscription, insofar as it redeploys stereotypes of the madwoman and her hysteria that could be considered aesthetically and ethically counterproductive. Beyond her reduction to a quasi-animal, the mother is also conceived as a quasi-hallucination in this scene, rendered immaterial to the point where the audience is invited to doubt her bodily existence. As Mum frog-hops around on the private side of the stage, Richard tells his Doctor about a time when he bumped into his mother in Russell Square, whereupon she began croaking like a frog. "But it was more kind of a self-willed apparition, really," says Richard (41). Two very different experiences are had here: on one side of the stage, the mother's guttural belching is a strong affective expression of embodiment; but on the other side, she is imaginatively disembodied, reduced to a quasi-hallucination.

According to feminist sound studies scholar Marie Thompson, the scream has historically been associated with irrationality, madness, hysteria, animality, excess, and "a lack of affective regulation" and, as such, the scream accompanies "imaginations of femininity at its most vulnerable" (151). Indeed, the mother's croaking slowly modulates into a scream, culminating in one final cry that actually distorts the microphone and rattles my ears—metaphorical excess becoming material. In reclaiming the scream away from primitivizing logic, Thompson argues that this vocalization is in fact a "trans-species mode of expression" adopted by many beings under duress; coincidentally, she gives the example of the horned frog tadpole, which lets out a high-pitched sound when threatened (152). For Thompson, the scream is thus an expression of refusal, of hope, and of "liveness in the face of death" (152). In this regard, the mother refuses to be silenced by her children and by the Doctor. The more she croaks and yells, the more they tell her to stop. "Look. Stop it. The doctor said," commands Rupert, to which Mum replies, "I can't stop" (43). Then, in a final act of refusal to be silenced, Mum tears down the curtains on the dividing wall, revealing her embodied self to the audience on the public side. This act of refusal also takes her frog croaking partly out of the cognitive realm of mental signification and into the corporeal realm of affective intensity.

The associations between the mother's noisiness and her gender remain a problem for the listener, however, because the scream is still deeply associated with female hysteria and lack of control. Returning to Carson's question about how one's listening is conditioned by one's presumptions about gender, I would suggest that the play reinforces the long-standing association between unruly vocality and femininity. For the same reason that we might ask why Richard has to ironically carry a carving knife, we might ask why the play has to portray the mother figure—the play's sole female—according to a pervasive trope of female excess and animality. In this instance, it becomes clear that the play's ethos of uncertainty does a disservice to its representation of female madness. If it were made clearer, in Thompson's sense, that noisiness is a natural response to being under duress, and not simply a symptomatic outburst, then we might hear such exchanges in a different register.

Mad Metaphor

The initial impulse behind this chapter came from noticing a tendency among theatre critics to ignore the metaphoricity of certain kinds of pseudo-mad experiences, suggesting that to put on headphones or to hear voices from behind a wall is to literally come to occupy another person's subjectivity, to hear as they hear and feel as they feel. In a broader sense, then, my overarching concern is with the limits of empathy, affect, and intersubjectivity. Though I believe that experimental theatrical forms can shift public perception around madness, at best reversing stigma and educating audiences, I think there is a tendency towards a kind of fetishistic disavowal—in Slavoj Žižek's sense of saying "I know very well [...] but nevertheless"—when we pretend that these virtual experiences have a more-than-metaphorical relationship to actual experiences (*Living* 9). Kane applies the disavowal formulation as such: "I know very well that the voice has a source, but nevertheless [when I close my eyes], I believe that it doesn't" (221). He calls this same mode of belief one of "acousmatic phantasmagoria" (221). For the acousmatic effect to be produced," says Kane, "the technical cause [...] is typically suppressed or taken out of consideration" (221). This act of suppression often involves a perceptual process of willfully ignoring the material and spatial conditions of a sound so as to bolster some kind of fantasy, privileging the aforementioned transcendental over the mundane (116). In *Eradication*, what is mundane is the fact that audience members very likely go into this production knowing about the whole hallucination conceit; moreover, we know that there are people on the far side of the wall making these noises. When your roommate calls out to you from the next room, for instance, you would not call that an auditory hallucination. And yet, many of us have also sworn that we heard or felt a phantom phone buzz. Auditory hallucination, then, may indeed be "the basic fact of mental life," as Robin Mackay argues, but its factuality does not mean that phantasmagoria can simply be manufactured on a whim (12). In a fundamental sense, then, simulatory modes of representation rely on a denial of the acousmatic.

If the acousmatic veil, as Kane suggests, has operated as a kind of fetishistic screen onto which we project our fantasies, then *Eradication*'s dividing wall, as a sound object, serves to fetishize a number of things, including auditory hallucinations, madness simulations, and—somewhat more awkwardly—empathy and intersubjectivity. As of June 2017, the disabled activist Arielle Silverman, talking about disability simulations, has said that "more research on this topic is badly needed" (par. 2). Citing Mark Riccobono, who is the president of the National Federation of the Blind, Silverman suggests that there is an important difference between simulations that provoke fear versus those that provide useful information (par. 2). In fear-provoking simulations more emphasis is put on communicating hardship and the "plight of disability" (par. 5). To the extent that Ridiculusmus's sound design emphasizes a sense of confusion, they run the risk of intensifying "people's preexisting fears and misconceptions" about schizophrenia and psychosis (par. 6). Simulations, in other words, have the potential to confirm those horrors wrought of misunderstanding. As Tanya Titchkosky, Devon Healey, and Rod Michalko put it, when simulations assume a normative position from which spectators and auditors imaginatively diverge, not only is disability framed as either lack or excess, but temporary blindfolds, wheelchairs, and earplugs can encourage someone to ask the wrong questions about sightedness or able-bodiedness or soundness of mind. That is, "Can there be anything more horrific than the lack of such a gift or the possibility of losing it?" (134).

Though Silverman writes about simulations in the context of social psychology, this problem is equally under-considered in theatre and performance. Theatre practitioners, I argue, need to engage with the problems of simulation in order to support more thoughtful representational practices and politics around madness. The first step towards such goals would be to ask how madness simulations actually function in plays such as *Eradication*. As per Silverman's critique, some simulations employ more oblique analogies than others. She deems backwards text, for example, a "crude dyslexia simulation" (par. 4). We should be careful, however, not to pursue a sense of fidelity to mad perception, striving for phenomenological accuracy, since this only leads to deeper essentialism, trying to perfect an imperfectible representation. More importantly, following Silverman, we should ask questions about such simulations, rather than take them for granted. Following important work by disability scholars such as David T. Mitchell and Sharon L. Snyder, we should treat metaphors with due suspicion, since this is the domain in which harmful stereotypes and general misunderstandings often proliferate. As per Mitchell and Snyder, corporeal metaphors imbue narratives with a sense of materiality, with the disabled body becoming a convenient symbol of abstract qualities such as villainous corruption, marshalling "simplistic associations between exterior form and psychic disposition" (112). Something similar seems to be at play in the transformation of psychic experience into formal sound design choices. In this case, the metaphors are more often immaterial. Disembodiment, in the form of veiled actors on the far side of the stage, for example, helps deliver "the symbolic potency of the message"—the message, in this case, being: this is what it is like to experience auditory hallucinations (64). Though the disabled body is often "an overdetermined symbolic surface" in these scholars' estimation, this play relies heavily on under-determining the body so as to make mock auditory hallucinations seem more real (64). In other words, it is necessary that the actors be invisible for the simulation to work its magic. Indeed, Kane suggests that this dynamic of absent presences is fundamental to the acousmatic listening situation: "One central, replicated feature of acousmatic listening appears to be that under-determination of the sonic source encourages imaginative supplementation" (9).

Perhaps this notion of "imaginative supplementation" offers us a more nuanced way of thinking about the play's sensory effects, since it invites us to ask about the nuanced analogical operations at play in the so-called replication of auditory hallucinations. What are the specifics of the phenomenal analogy whereby some but not all members of the audience might experience something akin to a hallucination? What does the form and protocol of the play do—and emphatically *not* do—in terms of dramatizing this analogy? How does the play's use of sound highlight the provisionality of one's own listening position? By what formal means does it attempt to transmit mad auralities or, in other words, to promote listening-as-other? Finally, is the simulation understood analogically or empirically (in terms of its "accuracy")?

All of these questions point towards what I am calling, somewhat clunkily, a mad phenomenal analogy, which departs from lived experience of mad phenomenology. Ridiculusmus's play, I contend, is not interested in the operations of phenomenology at a subjective level. Rather, it treats so-called auditory hallucinations mechanistically, as though controlling the objective sonic world can reproduce this aural experience *en masse*.[6] This view of phenomenology is heavily divorced from narrative and lived experience. Yet, Eleanor Longden and Philip Thomas have suggested that narrative identity is fundamental to mad phenomenology. Voice hearing, these authors tell us, should be thought of as historical, causal, and contextual; without narrative, we are simply left with "phenomena divorced from the contexts of the lives that hold those experiences." (188). Longden and Thomas reject the "abnormal perception" account of psychosis and, recalling Mackay's proposition that hallucination is a "basic fact of mental life," they argue that voice hearing is a "normal human variation" (189). Schizophrenia, for these authors, is a "putative, decontextualized illness" (189). I call this play's relationship to schizophrenia and psychosis one of a mad phenomenal analogy because if, following Longden and Thomas, voice hearing involves "faulty attributions of self-generated events to external sources," then *Eradication* does the opposite in making faulty attributions of externally-generated events to the self (190).

The dividing wall itself is one of the primary instruments of this analogy, since it externalizes dissociation by dividing the room in two and, in so doing, allows audience members to metaphorically experience the non-self (actors on the far side of the wall) as the self (those actors' voices, allegedly heard inside audience members' heads). Ironically, such analogies are not "phenomenal" in the evaluative sense; indeed, they are often less than. For better or for worse, mad phenomenal analogies are the engines of madness simulations. They are the "simulation tools" as described by the research psychiatrists Shuntaro Ando, Sarah Clement, Elizabeth Alexandra Barley, and Graham Thornicroft in their systematic review of hallucination simulations (8). Though these tools may promote some level of understanding, as such studies have shown, "simulated hallucinations have contradictory effects on stigma, increasing empathy but also the desire for social distance" (8). Given that medical professionals themselves are just recently, within the past decade, starting to ask questions about psychiatric simulations, this ought to be a bigger point of consideration within the ongoing empathetic turn in theatre, wherein a cottage industry is being built around relating experiences of alterity to paying audiences. From the total theatre of Peter Brook's *Marat/Sade* (1963), to Andy Houston's site specific tours of a Saskatchewan asylum in *The Weyburn Project* (2002), to Shannon Yee's immersive hospital experience, *Reassembled, Slightly Askew* (2014), to Pussy Riot's immersive prison experience, *Inside Pussy Riot* (2017), to the After Hours Theatre Company's immersive asylum experience, *One Flew Over the Cuckoo's Nest* (2018), there have been many productions over the past few decades that make use of psychiatric simulations. *Eradication* joins this list of shows within the wider experience economy that offer audience members a kind of psychiatric tourism. In the next section, I discuss the relationship of simulation to mimesis, and "the criticism that disability simulations provide an unrealistic experience," though the psychiatric realism question turns out to be something of a red herring (8). At this point, I should reiterate my position that such simulations should not be *more realistic*. By stressing the metaphoricity of simulation, what I actually want to communicate is that the discourse around representing mad auralities is actually too invested in the question of fidelity, to the point of making false promises to the listener.

Mad Mimesis

Looking beyond the production itself, it is worth noting how often write-ups about *Eradiction* use the language of simulation. Reviewers such as Laura Barnett in the *Guardian* have said that the show "replicates the experience of having an auditory hallucination" (n.pag). Again and again, the discourse surrounding this play's reception returns to the idea of replication, simulation, and mimesis. Another reviewer of the play, Tim Read, suggests that the company's "approach to staging brings an audience about as close to the reality of mental illness as it is possible to get," as if to forget that people actually live inside that reality ("Civilian Theatre" n.pag). One starts to notice what I mean here with regards to the overassertive rhetoric surrounding the play. Note, in particular, the reviewer's implicit assumption that mental illness is something that just happens inside a brain, independent of social context. This is precisely the problem that Longden and Thomas acknowledge when they say that so-called objective phenomena cannot be detached from subjective, lived experiences (188). Along similar lines, Tanya Titchkosky, Devon Healey, and Rod Michalko suggest that the logics of simulation can make it seem as though "the meaning of disability resides in the nature of an impairment and need not be understood as culturally produced" (128).

The presumed mad mimesis of this play witnesses a consistent jump in logic from experiencing mock-hallucinatory sounds to experiencing psychosis to experiencing what it is like to live with so-called schizophrenia, which is an issue unto itself because the symptom of voice hearing is not universal to the diagnostic category. Aural mimesis poses further complications because, being a secondary sense for most, it is more likely to be taken for granted, just as the reviewer quoted above has done. To begin with, the notion that this play, a fiction, would bring the audience as close as possible to the reality of mental illness is a peculiar oxymoron, and one that presumes that the audience is inherently positioned *outside* of madness. Meanwhile, it is unclear what precisely "reality" refers to, whether lived experience as a whole, or sensory awareness in particular, or perhaps simply hardship in the empathic sense. In any case, such statements reinforce my apprehension that those artistic strategies which propose to bring us closer can often move us further away, creating more distance and potentially a false sense of understanding.

Sound alone carries much of the persuasive power here, especially in combination with all of the mystifications that surround immersion and the bold promises of the experience economy.[7] When the desired outcome is to get "as close to the reality of mental illness as it is possible to get"—which surely must be read in terms of desire and not just theatrical effects—and when that closeness has an ethical component in terms of increasing empathy, there is all the more reason to ignore the messy essence of mimesis. As Lynne Kendrick notes, sound is often "considered to be actual" because it "invites us into an aural present which is often associated with encounter, interiority and immersivity" (42). In the case of *Eradication*, the audience is invited into all of these modes of relation simultaneously via sound: an encounter with madness, a peek into the interiority of the other, and immersion within a mad frame of reference.

It is not just the critics, however, that speak in such hyperbolic terms. On the company's website, for example, Ridiculusmus describes "an audience split in two experiencing auditory hallucinations" (cover copy). Not "experiencing what it is like" or "experiencing something formally analogous to" but simply "experiencing." This raises the thorny question as to what actually "counts" as a so-called hallucination, and whether the audience is meant to experience said hallucinations uniformly, with no individual perceptual differences. Here, I should clarify that I am not arguing for an essentialized understanding of psychosis or schizophrenia in trying to determine what constitutes a legitimate experience of hallucination. Indeed, as François J. Bonnet says, "the spectrum of hallucinated sound is broad and gradated" (173). Be that as it may, I wonder if this is a responsible or nuanced enough way of describing how individual audience members perceive sound and madness in this play.

Take, for example, the following reviewer at the *Times* who says that the production's perceptual programming—its attempts to convey mad aural mimesis—was thwarted by its ambiguous sound design: Kate Bassett describes "awkward pauses as [the actors] wait for intercut lines from over the wall, many of which are barely audible" (par. 4). In a moment of cheeky insightfulness, Bassett adds: "This is, inappropriately, a case of not hearing voices clearly enough" (par. 4). Though the production encourages "polyphony" and "tolerance of uncertainty," the reviewer calls these "buzzwords"—no doubt as a result of her frustrating listening experience (par. 1). Such thwartings are integral to any kind of rigorous phenomenology that would account for individual perceptual differences. Bassett's account of an aurally strenuous evening at the theatre brings to the foreground the problem of assuming a universal listening subject. The logics of simulatory hallucinations and mad aural mimesis most explicitly fail to account for deaf and hard-of-hearing audience members. But these logics also fail to account for genuine accounts of mad listening. One of the major internal contradictions of Ridiculusmus's sonic dramaturgy is that it trumpets tolerance of uncertainty at the same time as it attempts to simulate hallucinations for every audience member, whereas proper uncertainty would have to allow for momentary breakdowns within the production's sonic regime, as described by Bassett.

Zooming out momentarily, it is worth noting that the concept of mimetic sound has a long history. The classicist Stephen Halliwell tells us that one of the first known descriptions of mimesis referred to a choral performance from 600 B.C. in which a chorus of maidens was said to "bewitch its audiences by the performance of hymns" and could represent "the voices of all men and, literally, the sound of castanets," leading some audience members to imagine that they heard their own voices among the maidens (18). Clearly *Eradication* is not the first play to tap into the bewitching power of aural mimesis. Other terms, such as "sonic mimesis" and "audio mimesis" and "auditory mimesis" have been widely used outside any singular theoretical context, from literary analysis to audio engineering to sound studies more recently. I prefer "aural" as a qualifier because it implicates the listener's perception in the representational dynamic. Aural mimesis has manifold histories, from the invention of the phonograph, which Douglas Kahn calls "the mimesis machine" (70) to Filippo Tommaso Marinetti's "notion of onomatopoeia standing for the oral/aural *mimesis* of the world," as articulated by Mladen Ovadija (6). In the next section, I consider another long-standing correlation—namely: the entwining of mimesis with the concept of intersubjectivity, and the ways in which sonic realism leads us to think that we are getting a true-to-life experience of the other.

Radical Difference and Imaginative Sameness

Since much of the company's work is focused on combating stigma and depathologizing schizophrenia, it makes sense that Ridiculusmus would want to highlight the latent hallucinatory potential in all people. This move towards undermining sanism through universalization might be politically productive, but it also threatens to flatten out differences. On this issue, Peggy Phelan finds a third way between identity and post-identity politics by insisting on the "both/and" standpoint of post-structuralism. "It is possible," she says, "to see everyone as disabled, while also and at the same time recognizing that there are conceptual and perceptual frames that interpret specific events and specific bodies as extraordinary" (324). As such, it is important to insist on specific material differences in people's experiences, though those experiences may, to some extent, be analogous.

As Anna Harpin says, "starting with a radical embrace of difference" may be more productive than appealing to "imaginative sameness" (103). Must we feign the symptoms of a condition to empathize with it? As discussed above with reference to Brian Kane's analysis of the Pythagorean veil, perhaps what appears to be a more empathetic form of listening is in many cases just another form of fetishism, especially in those instances where audiences are promised a mad sensory experience. How, then, can we discuss aural subjectivity in non-universal and non-essentialist terms and enact what Harpin calls "empathy without sameness" (103)?

Consequently, can we imagine intersubjectivity without sameness? The concept of intersubjectivity takes multiple shapes within a sound studies context. Following Shannon Yee, Susan Bennett describes "intersensorial processing" as the means by which performers and audience members share a common headspace (1943). Describing her own piece of immersive headphone theatre, *Reassembled Slightly Askew*, and how it communicates the experience of brain injury, Yee remarks that "it's one step better than walking in somebody else's shoes. It's getting inside somebody's head and allowing an über-first-person perspective of the hidden disability" (McNay, "Shannon Yee"). Compare Yee's remark to that of Read, the reviewer, above, who said that *Eradication* brings us as close as possible to the reality of mental illness. When we are talking about immersive theatre—loosely defined— we are often talking about a mode of "über" relationality. In fact, Yee and Read are essentially saying the same thing. The "über" purports to bring us closer and closer until we are in the ever-receding horizon of an über-first-person. But the question remains: can we actually move any closer to the other's experience than we were before—before the binaural headphone technology and immersiveness as a construct? Or did the über-first-person peak with, say, the nineteenth-century novel?

For philosopher Dan Zahavi, "the question [...] is whether simulation will ever allow for a true understanding of the other or will it merely let me attain an understanding of myself in a different situation" (*Phenomenological Mind* 197). Put this question to *Eradication* and it sounds like this: will simulations ever allow me to know what the lived experience of voice hearing is like, or will it merely allow me to experience my own hallucinatory potential? Simulation theory finds purchase in multiple contemporary theories of intersubjectivity, including kinaesthetic empathy, wherein we are said to imaginatively reproduce, via mirror neurons, the embodied actions of performers and thus come to share their experience in some way. Maurice Merleau-Ponty articulates this as such: "No sooner has my gaze fallen upon a living body in the process of acting than the objects surrounding it immediately take on a fresh layer of significance; they are no longer simply what I myself could make of them, they are what this other pattern of behaviour is about to make of them" (*Phenomenology* 412). The problem with kinaesthetic empathy, as with sonic empathy—and as with all forms of what philosopher Peter Goldie calls "empathetic perspective-shifting"—is that "fellow-feeling is not susceptible to ambitious projects" (*Empathy* 9). In other words, a production such as *Eradication* cannot simply provoke an empathy response in a top-down manner. Some room must be left for failures of empathy and thwartings of intersubjective identification, as is evident in Bassett's review of the play, which demonstrates the ways in which simulations are vulnerable to even the slightest awkwardness.

There is perhaps, however, an inherent awkwardness in the asymptotic nature of the simulation—its inability to access the thing in itself. Speaking to the problems that empiricism demonstrates when faced with unexplainable phenomena, Merleau-Ponty suggests that "intellectualist reflection" upon unfamiliar modes of consciousness will typically "construct the hallucinatory phenomenon instead of living it" (*Phenomenology* 392). "We must stop constructing hallucination," he adds, "or indeed consciousness generally, according to a certain essence" (392). For Merleau-Ponty, there is always an element of consciousness held within "an invisible reserve" (*Visible* 152) that exterior perspectives cannot access—a "private world" that may have "close correspondence" with what others hear and see, but which is nonetheless closed off from "the other's lived experience"—and yet, he suggests that the common world between people prevents total solipsism, since it exceeds any single frame of reference (10).[8] Perhaps most applicable to the play in question is Merleau-Ponty's position on shared perspectives:

> What is being sought is not a fictitious coincidence of myself and others, of my present self with its past, of the doctor with the patient; we cannot take over another person's situation, relive the past in its reality, or illness as it is lived through by the patient. The consciousness of others, the past, or illness, can never be brought down in their existence to what I know of them [...] I am sitting before my subject and chatting with him; he is trying to describe to me what he 'sees' and what he 'hears'; it is not a question either of taking him at his word, or of reducing his experiences to mine, or coinciding with him, or sticking to my own point of view, but of making explicit my experience, and also his experience as it is conveyed to me in my own [...] and to understand one through the other. (*Phenomenology* 393)

For the purposes of this study, Merleau-Ponty's theories are useful for grappling with the problems of analogy and simulation. On one side, the philosopher contends that "the imaginary is not an absolute inobservable: it finds in the body analogues of itself that incarnate it" (*Visible* 77). On the other side, he acknowledges that "I do not have that private landscape as I have my own" and that one's perspective is "always divergent" from another person's (78). This strikes me as true of *Eradication*, where the audience maintains intellectual distance from the lived experience of voice hearing, as embodied in an actual person. The inner realities that Ridiculusmus stages are pure exterior, pure simulation. In phenomenological terms, it is the equivalent of an ethical encounter with a hologram. How, in such a context, can an audience be said to empathize with an absent subject? When we empathize with an actor performing madness, what exactly are we empathizing with? While attending to the simulatory framework of *Eradication*, the audience is, in *Merleau-Ponty*'s sense, made to feel as though "we are two witnesses capable of hovering over the same true object, or at least of exchanging our situations relative to it" (13). However, it is this very quest for simulatory logic—an "unjustifiable certitude" in accessing the thing in itself—that ultimately "brings us back to the dilemmas" (11).

Conclusion

This chapter has aimed to demonstrate that *Eradication* does not stage mad listening so much as it stages acousmatic listening, and that fidelity-based simulations of mad listening are untenable for the same reason as are simulations of normative listening. Following Kane, I am wary of pre-given ontologies of the sort that Woods and Haynes advance when they say they intend to provide the audience with an experience of auditory hallucinations, as best they can ("Inside" 05:30–05:55). For Kane, the acousmatic situation is "agnostic" about its potential modes of listening. Even though it is an acousmatic play that prizes tolerance of uncertainty, *Eradication* shows an irreconcilable commitment to a pre-given—and thus hardly agnostic—mode of listening. If mad auralities were to be simulated at an imaginary endpoint within the fidelity model, it could not be within the safe space of the theatre to begin with, under which conditions the experience is granted a level of acceptability that it does not often have beyond these walls.

Writing about Lodge Kerrigan's 1993 film *Clean Shaven*, which uses a number of filmic techniques to depict psychosis, mad studies scholar Anna Harpin makes a number of important distinctions that might help bring this discussion to a close. She writes:

> In placing an audience, then, temporarily in the 'unthinkable' space of psychosis, Kerrigan does not imply one now *knows* schizophrenia. Instead, he simply makes room to affectively consider the practices whereby one attempts to *understand* another's experience. The incompleteness of this gesture in *Clean, Shaven* signals his desire to de-situate the relationship between knowledge and empathy. And here an audience thinks *with* not *about* the atmosphere of profound paranoia. (206)

Contrast this sentiment with descriptions of *Eradication*, drawn from medical professionals at the 2013 Dialogic Conference in Finland. These professionals suggest that the play is "different," "fruitful," and "realistic" ("Responses"). The idea of "fruitfulness" is especially pertinent here, because it highlights the utilitarian aspect of so-called mental health plays—the idea that they should have specific outcomes such as improving standards of care, making audience members more knowledgeable and medical professionals more professional. Though I disagree with Harpin when she says that listening *with* is more productive than listening *to* (I think both have their own representational problems), she is right to insist on a difference between knowledge and understanding. In this regard, perhaps it would be better to conceive of stigma-busting theatre—as *Eradication* valiantly attempts to be—not in terms of learning but of unlearning. According to Harpin, representations always partly falsify experience (174). Though I have noted a few examples of falsified experience in this chapter, I want to reemphasize once again that my primary research objective is not to determine the authenticity of madness representations, and their degree of proximity to lived experience, as if to suggest that the distance is improvable, or that these simulations could be perfected until they achieve their intended effects. Rather, at most I wish to give formal context and descriptive language to unchecked assumptions. If simulation is aimed at knowing, then I have been arguing for the opposite. Kuppers's "radical unknowability" (88) and Harpin's "radical embrace of difference" (103) might therefore require a radical gesture aimed towards more closely engaging with the role of the veil, the wall, and other such structures that play host to our projections.

In *Immaterial Bodies: Affect, Embodiment, Mediation* (2012), Lisa Blackman observes that "psychic phenomena have always been technical, modulated and mediated through particular techniques" and have also been historically "bound up with particular fantasies" such as the "the desire for complete sympathetic union with the mind of another," which Pamela Thurschwell calls an "erotics of mind" (73). Such fantasies require that the mind be "porous and permeable to the other and not bound by structural constraints" (73). The next chapter turns to another set of structural constraints that uphold the very same fantasy via other technological, affective, and aesthetic means. The "problem of telepathy" or "mental touch" or "mimetic communication" as Blackman variously calls it, takes on different shape in the context of headphone theatre, for example, where something as literal as the proximity of an audio source plays a significant role in enacting the fantasy of mind-melding. Through a comparative analysis, the next chapter thus moves closer to the supposed site of exchange, i.e., the boundaried psyche and its oft-disembodied representation in performance.

Notes

1. This chapter works closely with two contested terms: "auditory hallucination" and "schizophrenia." According to Eleanor Longden, a research psychologist, and Philip Thomas, a psychiatrist in the

United Kingdom's National Health Services, the first of these is considered "depreciatory" and pathologizing, and the second is "best avoided because it has no construct validity, and thus its etiology has yet to be established" (190). The preferred terms would be "voice hearing" and "madness," respectively. If, in this chapter, I use the contested rather than the preferred terms, it is only because they reflect the discursive context of my analysis (i.e., these are the terms used by the majority of my case study's interlocutors. A thorough evaluation of these terminological differences is beyond the scope of this chapter, however).

2. By interlocutors, I refer to a range of critical discourse from reviews to academic analysis, which represent a spectrum of interpretive contexts. No doubt, public and scholarly reception reflect very different levels of critical engagement; however, by marshaling a full range of responses, I hope to demonstrate some of the common presuppositions that underlie wider conversations about madness representation and simulatory aesthetics. These contexts are also distinct from discourse emerging from the production itself (advertisements, etc.) which is often hegemonically "imposed from above," as Scott Magelssen puts it (6).
3. In 2012, Gardner wrote something similar: "As new works plunge audiences into ever more extreme situations, there's greater need than ever for artists to consider the ethics of manipulation" ("Interactive" n.pag).
4. According to Lisa Blackman, "to listen, hear, or see through another's voice requires a different kind of technology of listening based on seeing through mediated forms of perception, or what [Grace] Cho (2008) terms an ethics of entanglement ("Embodiment and Voice Hearing" 307). The present study is explicitly concerned with these ethics in the context of *Eradication*, and the formal means by which mad listening is mediated.
5. In "What is a Sign?" (1894), Charles Sanders Peirce defines the indexical sign as one which shows "something about things, on account of their being physically connected with them. Such is a guidepost, which points down the road to be taken" (5). Hence, the sound of the pill bottle described above indexes (points to) "medicine".
6. It is this gesture toward *en masse* replication and reception that I describe as a problem of "universalization." To similar ends,

Scott Magelssen argues that one of the major potential problems of aging simulations is that they can sometimes, in the context of his analysis, "treat older Americans as a monolithic identity" without taking "other cultural factors into account such as race and ethnicity, gender and sexuality, class status, geographic region," and so on (154). This problem speaks to both the reification of madness through stereotypical characters, as well as the presumption of an ideal audience member, who purports to experience such simulations exactly as they are intended.

7. One consistent "promise" of immersive theatres of the sort I describe throughout this book includes that of ethically encountering and ontologically overlapping with other lived experiences. A particularly thorough and incisive commentary on this phenomenon can be found in Natalie Alvarez's *Immersions in Cultural Difference: Tourism, War, Performance* (2018), where the author analyzes a variety of troubling immersive productions, including an immersive simulation of a terrorist training camp, and a fictional Mexico-US border run, designed to promote "a deeper understanding of and intimacy with the cultural others they stage" (9). Similar productions are detailed in Scott Magelssen's *Simming: Participatory Performance and the Making of Meaning* (2014).
8. Merleau-Ponty advances the metaphorical concept of the "chiasm" to describe a kind of exchange between self, other, and world. The analogy he provides is that of a glove turned inside out. Even though one sees "the wrong side of the glove," one is still able to infer its opposite configuration (*Visible* 263). Put another way: "The chiasm, reversibility, is the idea that every perception is doubled with a counter-perception" (264). As such, the object is never fully given, but exists at the ambiguous centre of multiple vantage points (or listening points, for our purposes).

CHAPTER 3

Mediated Mindscapes: On Staging Acoustic Interiority in Katie Mitchell's *Ophelia's Zimmer* and Janet Cardiff's *Her Long Black Hair*

Normative approaches to representing gendered madness have also tended to render women's distress legible, stable, and coherent: the hysteric faints, the murderess commits suicide, and the mad romantic sings unsound songs. According to theatre studies scholar Bridget Escolme, mad women have historically been confined to an "ordered and authorized space," depicted as unknowable and incoherent or deemed irrational and excessive (181). Discussing Ophelia's singing in relation to her madness, English Renaissance music and poetry scholar Leslie C. Dunn says that "critics tend to stress the visual and verbal signs of her distraction," though another line of interpretation could be that Ophelia plays up these signs with a sense of irony and cynicism (51). Dunn frames her own study within "the 'representational bonds' between gender, sexuality, and madness," as articulated in Elaine Showalter's foundational feminist study of Ophelia. She argues that the character is a "figure of song" whose unruly self-expression resists the logocentric and patriarchal order of speech (52). In 1997, Dunn noted that "Ophelia's singing has received short shrift in *Hamlet* criticism" (51). Today, this short-shrifting is perhaps truer of Ophelia's *listening*.

Two contemporary performance works, Janet Cardiff's *Her Long Black Hair* (2004) and Katie Mitchell's *Ophelia's Zimmer* (2015), reposition

M. Tomkinson, *Sound and Sense in Contemporary Theatre*, https://doi.org/10.1007/978-3-031-78034-9_3

the mad woman at the aural centre of the drama, using innovative sound design techniques. Both are well-documented and well-reviewed productions of significance for mad and feminist representation. The former was commissioned by New York's Public Art Fund and sponsored by Bloomberg, and the latter is a follow-up to playwright Alice Birch's hugely successful production of *Revolt. She Said. Revolt Again* (2014), commissioned by the Royal Shakespeare Company and staged internationally. The latter performance also arrived just a few years after Mitchell directed a video installation called *Five Truths* (2011) in which Ophelia's mad/death scenes are rendered in five different performance styles (Konstantin Stanislavski, Bertolt Brecht, Peter Brook, Antonin Artaud, and Jerzy Grotowski). This video work was commissioned by London's Victoria and Albert Museum in partnership with the National Theatre and can be found on YouTube with over 100,000 views. As evidenced by this level of patronage and engagement, the two plays under consideration in this chapter have notable reach and relevance. After its premiere, *Ophelia's Zimmer* quickly became a flashpoint for artistic and scholarly conversation, as the numerous reviews I engage with throughout this chapter will attest to; meanwhile, *Her Long Black Hair* remains an active critical touchstone in feminist criticism, sound studies, and beyond, with multiple publications revisiting the work over the past few years.[1]

Like Mitchell's *Five Truths* installation, this chapter compares disparate approaches to representing mad women. Formally, the plays under consideration are very different: the first (*HLBH*, henceforth) is a headphone-based audio walk that takes place throughout Central Park in Manhattan, whereas the second (*OZ*, henceforth) takes place on a traditional stage at the Schaubühne am Lehniner Platz in Berlin, where Foley artists provide a live soundtrack to Ophelia's isolation within a large glass box.[2] Beyond certain thematic overlaps—especially that of "immersion"—these two works reveal substantially different ways of staging mad auralities. By putting them in dialogue, I propose that we might get a better sense of their mechanics and political consequences through the concept of acoustic interiority, which Adrian Curtin defines as "sound that seems to come from 'within'" (25).

This chapter focuses on perceptions, discourses, technologies, and spaces of listening, asking how these variables inflect one's sensory experience of mad-sonic representation. Throughout, I address a variety of claims about simulatory modes of listening, as understood in specific listening contexts, such as the audio walk. These two performances serve as useful case studies for comparative analysis, insofar as they present distinct modes of simulation, one of which relies upon headphones to imaginatively reproduce interior space, whereas the other uses live sound design to approximate the protagonist's environment. In this regard, these two works serve as contrasting sites to explicate the representational strategies and issues at stake in trying to replicate mad auralities. Again and again, I am drawn to the question of intersubjective listening, or what I referred to in the previous chapter—with reference to Lisa Blackman's research—as "the problem of telepathy" (54). How, in other words, is the audience compelled to listen "with" a character, or from the narrator's point of audition? What are the dramaturgical means by which these performances convey mad subjectivity through sound? Finally, how do auditors actually engage with these sounds in practice, outside of given norms and ideals for listening?

Not only is it my goal to raise the volume on the heretofore unexamined aspects of these works, but I also want to listen more closely to what has already been said. For this reason, I make a point to reference the critical discourse surrounding these productions, analysing rhetorics of sound and madness. I note that this discourse is, in many ways, already about listening outcomes, even if much of it remains undertheorized or implicit. Theatre and media scholars such as Anna Harpin and Laura Dorwart have identified in these works two contrasting approaches to mad representation spanning from problematic forensic pathologization (Mitchell's play) to anti-sanist disidentification (Cardiff's audio walk). As these critics would have it, the works in question operate at either end of a representational spectrum. On one side, Mitchell's production is said to perpetuate stereotypes of madness, or "normative scripts and taxonomies of feeling," as Harpin puts it (196). Conversely, Cardiff's audio walk resists compulsory able-mindedness "by way of intentional nonlinearity, fragmentation, and disruption" (Dorwart 7). In this chapter, I interrogate specific mechanics of sound in representing mad subjectivity within these two works. Moving alongside the aforementioned critiques of legibility, emotional taxonomies, and normative versus non-normative "conditions of spectatorship," I proceed from the standpoint of the aural, asking what conditions of listening prevail in Mitchell's and Cardiff's work (Harpin 196).

One such condition is that of "shared" experience, as conveyed through soundscapes representing interiority, immediacy, and mental access. Cardiff's audio walk has been said to privilege deviant ways of thinking while making it compulsory to "think mad," (14) in opposition to compulsory able-mindedness—and that the work in question creates a "site of imagination" that promotes "shared consciousness," "community-building," and solidarity with other "neurologically atypical individuals" (Dorwart 13). In some sense, Cardiff's audio walk is said to be a work that dramatizes the very extreme of shared experience, then, while Mitchell's production is a work that dramatizes the very opposite: *HLBH* immerses the audience in the centre of the action, and *OZ* immerses the performer at a remove. Both works call upon their audiences to listen for what goes on inside a person's head and how one relates to one's inner world or sense of acoustic interiority. But how exactly, I wonder, does this sharing happen on the level of sound design? How do we know when it is happening? How are assumptions about madness encoded in moments of aural identification with a fictional character? And how are interior worlds built out of sound? Sound studies scholar Adrian Curtin is one of few theatre critics to date to ponder this last question. In particular, I am curious about how we might proceed from Curtin's observation that "drama's fascination with imaginary sound—sound that seems to come from 'within'—is connected to particular kinds of auditory engagement" (25). Curtin goes on to ask another important question—namely: how do we make sense of aesthetic translations of inner sound? (54). Throughout this chapter, I pose this precise question to Cardiff's and Mitchell's work in order to explore the particular ways that these two artists stage acoustic interiority, and to unpack the aesthetic and political implications of their respective approaches.

Ophelia's Zimmer in Context

Ophelia's Zimmer premiered in December 2015 at the Schaubühne in Berlin and played again in May 2016 at the Royal Court Theatre, London, as a collaboration between the two theatres.[3] The play was written by Alice Birch, directed by Katie Mitchell, and designed by Chloe Lamford, with sound design by Max Pappenheim, though the artists' roles often overlapped and cross-pollinated (Harpin, "You Were" 199). One critic summarizes the performance thusly: "The play follows [Ophelia] through five stages of drowning. It is a fair bet that we are inside her feverish mind but that is not a certainty. In any event, during this process, very little happens" (Fisher n.pag). These quiet domestic scenes are clearly intended to invert and subvert the plot-heavy source text, exhorting the audience to focus on what originally happened offstage and was thereby deemed unworthy of sustained attention. Throughout the play, a maid delivers Hamlet's letters to Ophelia in the form of cassette tapes, which contain increasingly aggressive sexual content. One reviewer suggests that Ophelia's manipulation of the tape deck, through forwarding and reversing, serves a counter-hegemonic function, "asserting control over what Hamlet is allowed to say in her bedroom" ("The Key of It" n.pag). Though the play presents many such opportunities to read Mitchell's Ophelia as a newly-empowered character, there remains the fundamental paradox of her voicelessness. That is, in giving Hamlet so much verbal space to show how much verbal space he takes up, the play can only reinscribe Ophelia's perpetual erasure rather than move beyond it. Mitchell is not unaware of this problem, however, and in fact she explicitly calls the work a "study in powerlessness" ("Proben-Trailer").

Adding to the critical reception of this play, Escolme argues that a multitude of *Hamlet* adaptations, in their depictions of Ophelia, "overlook the disruptive potential of her unconfined, wandering excess" and end up perpetually restaging her imprisonment, thus recapitulating representational issues that originate with Shakespeare's Ophelia (Harpin and Foster, *Isolated Acts* 13). Harpin notes this tendency in *OZ*, wherein it is suggested that "depression is a fateful object that, once inherited, is beyond escape" ("You Were An O" 205). Her thesis, writ large, is much less forgiving. Harpin argues that Mitchell's production reinforces "myths of mental illness" and that her directorial practice "re-enacts orthodox psychiatry's tidying away of life's mess" (206). Somewhat ironically, the play has been described as "A new work exploring Ophelia, freed from Hamlet," despite the fact that the play's title character spends the duration of the performance inside a claustrophobic plexiglass box ("Royal Court Theatre").

Though Mitchell deromanticizes Ophelia's death, she nonetheless reduces her to a gazed-upon body. Somewhat crass in its morbid objectification, the play's official promotional material asks: "How does she go mad? And does she really die sliding comfortably into a stream covered in flowers as her boyfriend's mother reports? Or is there something more sinister and strange going on? And what does the bloated dead body of a young girl floating in a river really look like?" ("Ophelia's Room" 1).

This question is answered directly by a man's voiceover at the beginning of each of the play's five sections. At the top of the first section, he says: "Mund und Nasen Raum werden über Wasser gehalten. Das Opfer gibt kaum Geräusche von sich. Das Atmen ist erschwert" ("Mouth and nasal cavities are held above water. The victim makes hardly any sounds. Breathing is difficult"; 00:00:21–00:00:35). The play ends with Ophelia's "Klinischer Tod" ("clinical death"), and her drowning is described in the language of a coroner: "Das Opfer erleidet einen Herzstillstand. Die inneren Organe werden von der Sauerstoff und Sauerstoffzufuhr abgeschnitten. Nach fünf Minuten ohne Sauerstoff sterben Zellen des Gehirns ab" (The victim suffers a cardiac arrest. Internal organs are cut off from oxygen and oxygen supply. After five minutes without oxygen, brain cells die; 01:47:42–01:48:05).

Speaking to the play's medical luridness, Harpin reminds us that there is "no way to do madness 'right'" according to some kind of perfectly drawn pathology, but that such a forensic gaze can be limiting and damaging to the extent that it renders "mad women as void shapes" or "decipherable objects" (210). This critique underscores the main shortcoming of Mitchell's work, which one might call the perennial problem of reinscription. Rather than rebuild Ophelia's narrative and the patriarchal machine that drives it, she takes us inside that machine to experience it all the more intensely. In this regard, Harpin's criticisms could take a more nuanced position on Mitchell's irony, since the play is awash in it. The performance adopts forensic aesthetics in order to comment on them. Notably, Harpin defines forensic aesthetics as a side effect of realism—an "unreal rigidity" of representation, marked by "the absence of mess, the absence of uncertainty" ("You Were an O" 210). Furthermore, the narrator describes Ophelia as an "Opfer" (a "victim"), thereby exposing his ideological position; moreover, the title character is silenced in order to depict her silencing. With a certain amount of heavy-handedness, then, the play does not offer a correction so much as a diagnosis. I want to foreground this contradiction, since it turns out to be one of the major talking points in *OZ* criticism. See, for example, this response from a blogger who reiterates this problem with reference to the play's sound design:

> You—in the audience—are given another point of reference to look at almost all the time, seeing two men make all the sounds of walking and doors opening and closing. Perhaps, again, this is a comment about men *still* getting to make all the decisions, and all the big noises, but as such

> it seems to undermine the mission here to also expose and undermine patriarchal power. It feels instead like it reinscribes it; larger and different, somehow. ("Postcards from the Gods" n.pag)

To find more nuance within Mitchell's work, we might acknowledge those moments where the work serves as more than a measurement, where the diagnostic quality of the material is exceeded by its complex treatment of the title character, or where the soundscape works in subversive ways to reorient the audience towards a more critical perspective on the source text's dominant ideologies.

There has been a flurry of scholarly writing about Mitchell's work in recent years, but only a small number of thorough critical engagements with this play. A special issue of *Contemporary Theatre Review* in 2020 was devoted to the director, with contributions from theatre scholars the likes of Tom Cornford, Anna Harpin, and Benjamin Fowler, the latter of whom is Mitchell's preeminent surveyist and biographer. Some research has already been conducted on Mitchell's soundscapes, and a little has been written about the director's depictions of madness; however, it remains necessary to synthesize the two, since Harpin's work on *OZ*, though reliably brilliant, does not once use the word sound. Meanwhile, Maria Elisa Montironi's research discusses both madness and sound but does not combine these sites of analysis in a meaningful way.[4] Where the latter author does combine these two sites, it serves as a curt apology for the play's representational strategies rather than a balanced critique.

My argument in this chapter moves in the opposite direction, towards questioning Montironi's idea that Mitchell's sound design uncomplicatedly shares Ophelia's "earpoint."[5] Furthermore, I agree with Harpin when she says that the main issue with Mitchell's depiction of madness is that it "reasserts the idea that feeling and experience are sovereign and bounded within individuals, as opposed to being relational, unfixed, and porous" (195). Notions of intersubjective listening, as suggested by Montironi's use of the term "earpoint" (a troublesome concept that perpetuates audist assumptions about the ear) are thus part of the problem, though these arguments are no doubt well-intentioned and characterize a great deal of scholarship about theatrical sound's superpowers of relationality, empathy, and other-orientedness. The concept of a shared "earpoint" might be compelling if further developed; however, Montironi uses the word only once, without explicitly defining the perceptual mechanics at play. In their conversation about the core ideas of Mitchell's work, theatre scholars Kim Solga and Dan Rebellato suggest that the playwright's feminism, which she was reticent to disclose in her early career, is based on recuperating naturalist aesthetics within a new tradition (Fowler 8). They note that feminists have been uneasy about naturalism because it is often tied up with predictable outcomes and psychological determinism—an inevitable death, for example (52). One might say that this sense of inevitability is precisely what Harpin takes issue with in her criticism of *OZ*, since Mitchell's adaptation is just one of many in which Ophelia ends up in yet another box, however tinged with irony that box may be.

On the subject of space, Cornford brings us back to the problem of sharing a so-called earpoint: "Spaces," he says, "are always composed of relations from which we cannot escape and which exceed any attempt to make them cohere from a single perspective" (80). That Mitchell's work resists such collapsing of perspectives suggests a fundamental uneasiness with reductionism. As such, the play in question makes for an exemplary case study since it upholds values of nuance and complexity but also reveals certain inconsistencies and shadow zones in the director's representations of women's madness.

Close Listening: *Ophelia's Zimmer*

The play begins with the rumbling of sub-bass, and I am immediately aware of the fact that these low tones lack the embodied dimension of live sound. A man's voice (belonging to Renato Schuch, who doubles as Hamlet) describes Ophelia (played by Jenny König) as a swimmer flailing in the water—the first of the play's five stages of drowning, corresponding with five acts. From the outset, one is immersed in an atmosphere of doom-and-gloom madness. Now, another narrator, a woman's voice this time (implied to be Ophelia's mother, voiced by Jule Böwe) describes Ophelia's pale face as she puts on a black dress and stands still in a humming blue room. Both narrators' voices have an authoritarian quality, as though they are experimental psychologists speaking over an intercom to a subject in another room. A sudden beep, like that of a text-message notification, signals a shift from night to day. An unseen rooster crows off in the imagined distance. Ophelia hums to herself as she puts on rain boots. An audience member coughs as Ophelia runs up an imaginary set of stairs, provided by the Foley artists offstage in their plexiglass box. A maid (played by Iris Becher) enters the room to deliver flowers, and her eyes track Ophelia's imaginary footsteps as they crunch along an imaginary gravel path where the front row meets the stage.

Here, sound design and choreography work together to create a "collusion, or confusion, of psyche and soundscape," (16), in Curtin's sense of the acoustic imaginary, or what he called "fantasized hearing" (31). The maid swivels her gaze in a slow, full left-to-right motion while tracking Ophelia's Foley footsteps as if to over-assert the binaural spatial positioning of this imaginary sound. In a way, this gesture also sets up rules for engagement, teaching the audience how to track these sounds and how to move with them. A few more high-pitched "dings" later, and Ophelia returns. Meanwhile, I am annotating the video in split-screen mode, shuttling between text and image, pausing to think, looking up page numbers for my secondary sources, and continuing. Just now, as I am sitting and watching, Ophelia is sitting and reading, perched on the edge of her bed, which suggestively resembles the metal-framed beds of twentieth-century psychiatric wards and prisons, well-recognized by now as a madness trope.

There is something "off" about Ophelia's room, never mind the fictional framing devices such as the sunken floor and the plexiglass booths. Specifically, I mean, the anachronisms: a twenty-first-century door with a twentieth-century bed and nineteenth-century furnishings. Most suggestive, perhaps, is the fact that she uses an old boombox to play her tapes—a vintage two-in-one radio/cassette device from the 1980s. Depending on where one situates her historically, this Ophelia appears to be condemned to obsolescence, fossilized within a museum-like room, stuck in past symbolisms that prevent her from changing. These stage elements once again evoke Escolme's argument that Ophelia's re-confining, and her continued infantilization, has haunted a great majority of modern adaptations of Shakespeare's play. Writing about a number of recent productions—including the Brighton-based theatre company DreamThinkSpeak's adaptation of *Hamlet*, *The Rest is Silence* (2012), which also enclosed the cast within four glass walls—Escolme argues that many of them have "trapped her within a semiotics of pitiably banal, mad femininity" (180). Echoing Petra Kuppers' argument against "clear-cut images" and "representational certainties" (*Bodies on the Edge* 123), Escolme makes a strong case for avoiding this approach:

> It strikes me that many of the representations of Ophelia discussed here are striving to create representational certainty, whether because of the nineteenth-century desire to read Ophelia as something more than a

> tawdry theatrical figure, sexually exposed in her madness, or whether in an attempt to confine her—behind a shopping trolley, or in a wheelchair, or behind a screen. (180)

Nevertheless, Mitchell's Ophelia is confined to the past. Some modern flourishes to the room suggest that an attempt has been made to update her context, but that even these attempts have been met with resistance, as though even the director could not implement the necessary representational changes. Now, in the video, a muffled voice calls out her name and she exits through this modern door to retrieve a drink of warm tea in a vintage cup. Then she goes back to sitting on her bed, reading. Every action is punctuated by a tense, low-level ambience, as if to tease the possibility of silence, but instead polluting that possibility. Sub-bass tones act as filler, a kind of gravitational field within which cohere all the loosely distributed moments of the work. Shortly, a letter from Hamlet arrives via the maid in the form of a cassette tape in an envelope—another suggestive jumble of historical media, this mix of envelope and cassette. Ophelia walks over to the cassette deck and presses play. Hamlet tells her that thoughts of her death have rendered him sleepless and without appetite. He speaks of carrying an image of her in his mind as if to reduce her to a concept while she sits there full-bodied in this room, a living contradiction. Suddenly, I am being thrown out of the moment by someone coughing near the microphone being used to record the play. The noise is startlingly loud in contrast to the sound of the action on stage.

If my reader will permit some meta-theatrical commentary: I am now coming to sense a strange resonance between Ophelia's activities and my own. She stops and starts the tape at will, rewinding occasionally to listen again, and in my analysis of this footage, I am doing precisely the same thing on my computer. Her control over the tape deck, however, is evidently meant to be a subversive gesture. As one reviewer puts it, "Hamlet's tapes, which arrive relentlessly, are a powerful reminder of the luxury of speech and contemplation; a luxury that has not been afforded to Ophelia"; however, she rebels against these acts of aural domination by "fast-forwarding the tapes, pausing them and rewinding them, asserting control over what Hamlet is allowed to say in her bedroom, and therefore onstage" ("The Key of It" n.pag). Indeed, Hamlet's cassettes are full of sexually aggressive ramblings, discussing nothing but his horniness while objectifying Ophelia's body in the crudest terms. Theatre scholar Benjamin Fowler nonetheless reads the character's control over the boombox as a rejection or reinscription of these terms:

> Her control of rewind and fast-forward made perception tangible as she lipped along to tender passages she had memorised or wound past sections that bored her. When Hamlet's description of licking her cunt interrupted her sewing, she stopped the tape only to rewind and replay. König's inscrutable listening face didn't reveal stable meanings, but her rewind suggested a fascination and a production critically searching the minute dynamics of reception and response in a character (and from an actor, as we will see) who more commonly absorbs aggressive male energy without reply. (242)

We quickly found out, however, that Ophelia's control of the dial is a totally insufficient mode of reclaiming power. In fact, it is not very long before Laertes (played by Ulrich Hoppe) unplugs the radio and removes it from the room to hasten her decline. Such a gesture reveals that Ophelia's temporary status as DJ of Hamlet's words was only ever "one sanctioned form of self-assertion as a woman, quickly followed, as if in retribution, by her death," to quote Showalter (80). As such, I find it necessary to qualify the rewinding-as-rebellion interpretation in light of what happens to the radio in Ophelia's absence.

During this sequence, Ophelia adds another layer to her outfit (which she will continue to do until the end of the play, her movement getting more restricted with every additional item). Her control over the tape deck becomes similarly restricted until, eventually, the device operates by itself, as though possessed, playing Hamlet's voice in reverse even as no one's there to hold down the button (00:16:01–00:16:40). Writing about the concept of "radio madness," Carolyn Birdsall and Senta Siewert note that "following the domestication of radio, the medium was portrayed as potentially causing disturbances in female listeners, with the implication that their nerves could not handle the sensory input of radio's mediated voices" (29). Knowingly or unknowingly, Ophelia's use of the boombox is positioned within a history of media excess, of gendered listening and female-coded madness. Such listening "disturbances" arise when Ophelia steps away from the silent boombox and the tape of Hamlet's voice begins to play, with a will of its own, in reverse. The timbre of the recording has a haunted, chipmunk-like quality. In one sense, this scene reduces Hamlet's speech to pure gibberish—a kind of short-circuiting and radio-jamming of male aurality and its phallogocentrism. But heard another way, the phantasmagoric reversed speech serves as a sonic trope of madness, indicating to the audience that Ophelia is hearing voices, and not just any voice, but one that has been warped beyond comprehension. Does this say more about her as a listener or him as a speaker? Moreover, does this scene place more scrutiny on the condition of his speech or the condition of her mind? And are we listening to the tape as heard in the room, or the tape as heard internally, via hallucination, by Ophelia? In the words of Birdsall and Siewert, these representations do not just form around pathologies of listening, but "pathologies of media" (28).

In the replacement of letters with tapes, there is an implicit move from the presumed logic of writing to the presumed illogic of speech. In other words: the cassette is a mad-coded medium. As a form of obsolete media, the tape is doubly unsound, since it is subject to distortion and decay, as is the recording embedded on its surface. On the topic of mass media and its phantasmagoria, Mitchell's production finds an unlikely companion in a 1963 short story by Keith Laumer called "The Walls," as discussed in the media historian Jeffrey Sconce's book on "haunted media" (151). Set in the distant future, the story tells of a woman who is "slowly driven to madness by her husband's desire for an ever more constricting television system in the home," which eventually manifests as four full-length walls of glass, imprisoning her within a television-like room and causing her to experience "video-induced psychosis" (152). Laumer's story, as Sconce describes it, is about "the abandoned housewife whose existence becomes completely 'mediated' by television" (152). Similar ideas are behind Ophelia's imprisonment within a highly mediatized space and her "technologically-induced madness," to borrow a phrase from Birdsall and Siewert (29). As these scholars put it, "One of the key aspects in modern sound technologies that have been thematized in terms of the uncanny or insanity is that they separate the voice from the body, and the site of speaking from its listening context" (30). This is true on an anatomical level: reading is a process of subvocalizing speech within one's own body, and so to replace letters with cassettes is to remove Ophelia's ability to do even this much. One need not cite Marshall McLuhan to know that these two communication formats can run hot and cold, active and passive, and that the cassette tape, in this instance, perpetuates Ophelia's silence and immobility. Quoting the film theorist Michel Chion, Birdsall and Siewert suggest that the disembodied voice—Chion's *acousmêtre*—"lends itself to associations with […] mental disturbance" (31). They describe acousmatic sound as an "ongoing aesthetic strategy" of theatrical and cinematic soundscapes, used to "approximate mental disturbance and auditory hallucinations" for audiences (41). One of the central tropes of this approximation is glossolalia, or babbling voices, projected over the stereo to signify an auditory hallucination or internal speech. This kind of disembodied voice projects and externalizes the subject's mind onto the playback device (36). As such, the boombox becomes a means of representing acoustic interiority, a fantasy of shared listening subjectivity between performer and spectator-auditor. For hearing audiences, Hamlet's glossolalia is experienced, in some sense, *through* Ophelia as a means of transmitting her listening.

Literary scholar and posthumanist N. Katherine Hayles discusses the titular figure of Samuel Beckett's *Krapp's Last Tape* (1958) in terms that resonate with Mitchell and Birch's protagonist. As Krapp sits, immobile, and listens to recordings of his past self, his gesture of rewinding audiotape might be understood as a means of figuratively "escaping from the constructions that have defined him," much as Ophelia's rewinding can also be read as a subversive act (85). Indeed, Ophelia presses pause in the middle of Hamlet's to-be-or-not-to-be speech, no doubt the most defining line of the play. Hayles also offers up the compelling analogy of the "parasitic monologue," which refers to the ability of language to invade private spaces, including that of consciousness (87). This term aptly describes the intrusion of Hamlet's voice into Ophelia's room—and, indeed, the play's title reminds us that this is her space, despite constant violations of her privacy. At one point, Hamlet embodies this parasitism when he bursts into the room and starts dancing to Joy Division's "Love Will Tear Us Apart," blasted at an aggressively loud volume. Dancing unselfconsciously in a fog of irony, this Hamlet burlesques a certain kind of egocentric, tragic love. The classic anthemic angst of the song plays out in contrast to Ophelia's genuine suffering. Taking the song's "tearing apart" to its literal conclusion, he violently grabs and shakes Ophelia, pushing her into a chair, and forcing her to watch him throw his weight around the room in a self-absorbed trance.

This theme of parasitism is entwined with the play's dramatization of acoustic interiority, which Montironi has discussed in terms of the "ear-point." The author takes for granted, however, that *OZ* is a "rebellious composition" that represents the "cacophonic, imposing and invasive 'sounds' of patriarchy as perceived by Ophelia" and that the play's "soundscape is capable of denouncing the patriarchy even more effectively than both visual and linguistic elements" (135). Montironi suggests that the audience vicariously experiences Ophelia's "auditory captivation" and metaphorically drowns alongside her in a deluge of sound (143). For this scholar, the play's attempt to "disintegrate syntax" can be considered a "rebellious 'feminist composition,' in dissonance with Shakespeare's dialogue-centred play" (135). Another interpretation, however, might be that the play's radiophonic glossolalia also serves to pathologize the protagonist. Montironi argues that by "sharing Ophelia's acoustic world, spectators can fully tune into the character and better understand her subjugation" (133). Crucially, however, I want to suggest that we cannot approach "sharing" as a given, disregarding the complexities of mediatization, that is, the means by which the act of sharing is constructed. When mad voices such as Hamlet's glossolalia appear to emerge from "within" Ophelia, such that the audience presumes to hear from her subjective listening position, we are confronted with a number of questions. First, is it really possible to share an earpoint? Second, what representational work has to happen on stage to convince audiences of this possibility? Third, what are the representational stakes for a mad-feminist account of this process?

In particular, I worry that the supposedly liberatory gesture of a shared earpoint can peddle certain falsities—tropes, stereotypes, and other misrepresentations—like any other form of symbolic exchange. What, then, are the consequences of sharing a false understanding? If we are to share Ophelia's acoustic world, then it is still important to ask what makes up that world. Looking back at the first of my three questions above, I would suggest that the concept of a shared earpoint does not hold up, if only etymologically. For one thing, the shared ear is an Archimedean point, a hypothetical central position that requires a total absence of surrounding context. We cannot share an earpoint without sharing an ear, and this, of course, is impossible. Moreover, for the same reason that it is untenable to hold a theory of mind for a character, we could not share Ophelia's earpoint—even if we wanted to—so much as Jenny König's (the actress who plays her). Another issue altogether is that the material conditions of sound are never the same for performers and audience. Foley, in this instance, is a caricature of sound: where the playtext describes amplified "Foley water" lapping and trickling, for example, the actual substance remains a silent pool onstage (Montironi 142). In this way, some Foley sounds can be metonymic, where amplification turns small drops of water into bucketfuls or even oceans. To share an earpoint with Ophelia, then, would be to ignore that we are on opposite sides of the speakers.

Much more could be said by way of unpacking this concept, but I would like to point out just one more significant sticking point. Consider the fact that we as the audience are positioned in an empowered position, relative to Ophelia; spatially, we are afforded a panoramic view of the stage, including the sound booths where her acoustic world is constructed. According to Montironi, the play "defies ocularcentric theatre semiosis"; however, the very presence of bright fluorescent sound booths suggests that much of the play's dramatic irony rests entirely on the fact that we are invited to visually identify sound sources that Ophelia cannot. In technical terms, we might say that many of the play's noises are acousmatic for her, and non-acousmatic for us, though this is not true of every sound (e.g., Hamlet's voice). Ultimately, this dramatic irony speaks to the presence of two radically different points of view or points of audition. If anything, the production enacts the inverse listening situation by making the audience complicit in Ophelia's subjugation. We are aware, or should be, that she is presented as a lab rat in this play, and yet we fantasize about sharing her limited perspective. It must be asked: if the play's Foley artists represent a patriarchal force that's responsible for manufacturing and manipulating Ophelia's sensory landscape, then why should the listener assume that her earpoint (as represented) is trustworthy? Remember that these Foley artists do not just present the world *to* her, but also represent (to us) the world as it is *for* her. Should we not hesitate, then, to share an earpoint with this Ophelia? After all, she has very limited capacity for self-definition and very little access to the means of audio production—all of the speakers and none of the microphones. In short, I would argue that there are many ways in which Mitchell's production empowers and adds nuance to the title character, but that a shared earpoint is not one of them.

In an interview with theatre scholar Bryce Lease, Mitchell says that she has used Foley sound effects in the past to create "the more abstract aural experience of what it was to be inside each character's head" (254). She reiterates this sentiment in her book, *The Director's Craft: A Handbook for the Theatre*, with reference to cinema: "Sound is also used in film to create a subjective impression of what it is like to be inside a character's head" (87). Likewise, the play's sound designer, Max Pappenheim, says that certain repetitive sounds, such as the bells and the footsteps, "gave Ophelia's existence a structure/routine that helped us move inside her head"

(Montironi 148). These representational strategies for depicting acoustic interiority are most pronounced when Ophelia begins to hallucinate the sound of water dripping, minutes before it begins to pool onstage, corresponding with the moment when she is given pills to swallow (01:34:30). Ophelia then asks the other characters if they see or hear water and they say nothing, moving through the room as if nothing is amiss, even as their ankles slosh through real water. By comparison with the play's earlier hallucinations, this scene of dual misperception serves to complicate the play's mad characterization. If glossolalia appears as a well-worn trope of mad speech and mad listening, then the sound design here adds a layer of ambiguity. Foley water from offstage mingles with the sound of legs wading through water onstage. In this instance, Ophelia hears "imaginary" water that others cannot see, and then real (by my account) water floods the stage that others cannot feel. This complication of reality invites us to ask: who's mad here? When this question arises, one can be sure that the play is at its most open-ended—no doubt a valuable quality in the context of mad representation where certainties proliferate in the form of diagnoses and stereotypes. Though scholars such as Harpin argue that Mitchell portrays "feeling states as neatly definable," the director's work is perhaps not so neatly definable itself, not least of all because of the ironies of reinscription mentioned earlier (196). To an extent, any criticism of the play's sound design along political lines can always be deflected to the play's internal sound designers, the Foley artists who control Ophelia's soundscape at the same time as they control the audience's. Despite this, I generally agree with Harpin's descriptors of the play's representational strategies—stable, predictable, knowable, scientistic, individualistic, forensic, taxonomic—and I agree that the director "perpetuates a nihilistic vision of madness as catastrophe" (198). It has been my aim throughout this section to develop this argument further by focusing our attention on specific sound design techniques aimed at formally representing acoustic interiority—but I have also tried to entertain alternative perspectives, locating nuances within Mitchell's work where credit is due.

As an afternote, I would like to point out that the play also reveals a truth about imbalances in the audio profession. As the gender studies scholar Roshanak Kheshti suggests, "the era of the feminization of listening has shifted yet again. Women represent only a small fraction of audio engineers" (182). Though Birch, Lamford, and Mitchell are a formidable production team, the onstage and offstage sound crew are notably lacking in gender diversity. According to the ethnomusicologist Rebecca Lentjes, sonic patriarchy is perpetuated through unevenly distributed agency in sound creation: "To borrow Suzanne Cusick's terminology, perpetrators of sonic patriarchy exercise 'acoustical agency'—not (only) because they are the sound-making agents, but because they are using sound as an expression of their embodied, patriarchal, political agency" (n.pag). Following Kheshti, Lentjes theorizes sound "as a phallic force" and the ear as a sexualized organ, "to be penetrated" (n.pag). In such a dynamic, aural space is invaded, sound becomes non-consensual, women are harassed, and "female bodily identity is reduced to open ears and silenced voices" (n.pag).

It is much the same for Mitchell's Ophelia: she is quite literally a captive audience, whose intersecting madness, gender, and sexuality serve as multiple loci of control. The slippage I am referring to, between production and performance—a lack of acoustical agency both within and without—demonstrates one of the fundamental problems of recapitulation and reinscription as an adaptational strategy. As can readily be seen from a number of responses to this play, including my own, Mitchell misses the opportunity to stage effective sonic interventions that could change the representational landscape around madness. In the next section, I turn to one of Janet Cardiff's most celebrated audio walks, with a similar character at its core, to see if it offers more or less radical ways of engaging with these themes.

Her Long Black Hair in Context

Theatre and disability scholar Laura Dorwart describes *Her Long Black Hair* (2004) as a work that exemplifies the mad pride movement and presents listeners with a "disruptive" and "subversive" representation of Ophelia-as-narrator (4). However, as with numerous other representations of this character, including Mitchell's, this Ophelia is likewise "frozen" and lacks "the potential for true escape" (12). That this Ophelia walks freely throughout central park, however, and actively refuses silence through narration, suggests certain measures of freedom, and defies the carceral heritage to which Mitchell's Ophelia belongs more transparently.

By way of clarifying my own interpretation of the character, it is important to note that Cardiff's walk contains a swirl of uncertain identities, such that it is never quite clear whom we are listening alongside. Also important to note is that, unlike in Mitchell's production, the audience is not invited to listen through the protagonist's perspective, but through the narrator's. The narrator vacillates between the artist herself, a narrative persona, an Ophelia whose journey ends by the side of a lake, and an Eurydice who continuously follows someone else. As it were, this "someone else" is also uncertain. The narrator retraces the steps (as we retrace her steps) of a mysterious woman with long black hair, whose likeness appears in the photographs accompanying the walk. This protagonist around whom the walk centres are also many other things: a random woman whose photographs ended up in a pawn shop, a gender-swapped Orpheus who refuses to look back at us, and her own version of Ophelia and Eurydice. There are many allusions in *HLBH*, but none of them explicitly reference *Hamlet*. It is primarily on the basis of an implied drowning that we might read Cardiff's protagonist as an Ophelian character, whose disheveled hair has served, since the eighteenth century, as a metonym for archetypal feminine madness. If only for the sake of clearer comparison with Mitchell's work, I follow Dorwart in discussing these personages with reference to Shakespeare's character; however, the audio walk itself insists upon a greater sense of ambiguity with regard to its characterization. Accordingly, I use my best judgement in deciphering the most relevant allusions throughout the work.

It must be said that my immediate listening context, not unlike my engagement with Mitchell's video documentation, is at a great remove from the original space of reception. Cardiff's walk takes place throughout Central Park in New York, which I traverse via Google Street View for lack of a better option (recall that I began writing this amid the early days of the pandemic). The original soundwalk involved a designated CD player and set of headphones, along with a packet of photographs. I sit behind a computer screen, miles away, trying to piece together a walking tour from a seated position, as though performing telesurgery. One major discrepancy in my listening is the lack of a palimpsestic aspect to this incomplete experience: there is no clash, no messy sonic entanglement between real-world New York and headphone New York, no ambiguity between prerecorded events and live events, no "haunted milieu" in theatre scholar Eirini Nedelkopoulou's description (122). Indeed, Nedelkopoulou argues that *HLBH* operates through ecstasis, stepping out of oneself and filling in for the absent corporeality of Cardiff's disembodied narrator: "the physical presence of the audience completes and enables the mixed-media walks. The audience's participation [...] is not simply an instance of seeing, listening and strolling around the space, but an embodied experience" (122). She calls this dynamic a "chiasmic" exchange—one of overlapping or intertwinement, following the phenomenologist Maurice Merleau-Ponty. Unfortunately, there is nothing especially embodied or proprioceptive or haptic or chiasmic or haunted or messy or entangled about my experience of the work. I bring this to your attention so that any claims I make about a representational shortcoming in the work are not immediately attributable to this problem of insufficient context. Indeed, I am well aware of the phenomenological instability generated by the play of auditory insides and outsides in *HLBH* and acknowledge that this dynamic is fundamental to the work. One might argue, as philosopher Mirjam Schaub has, that a mix of live and prerecorded sounds "destabilizes the perceived world immensely" and that this destabilization is a crucial aspect of the play's invitation to think and listen madly (3). By disambiguating the experience, my aim is to focus exclusively on what can be said about the recording, without speculating on the walk itself or the highly idiosyncratic way in which I have experienced it.

One silver lining to my experiential distance, perhaps, is that I can focus in greater detail on the nuances of Cardiff's recording and its formal qualities. If my listening seems to misrepresent the multisensory context of the work, then it is worth noting how scholars and critics fail to agree on the precise duration of the walk, with reported walk times ranging from 35 minutes up to 40, 45, and as high as 60 (the official time is 46 minutes). For a piece that explores notions of temporality, it is curious to see such extreme relativity among audience members' experiences.

As mentioned above, *HLBH* was commissioned by New York City's Public Art Fund and sponsored by Bloomberg. It is widely considered a canonical work within the history of the audio walk—a history with which Cardiff's name is synonymous, as is that of her partner George Bures Miller, who produced this piece. The walk had two runs (so to speak) during the summer of 2004 and 2005 but is now widely available online as a recording that people can download and take to the park on their own. Originally, the recording lived on CD players, which were distributed to participants at kiosks on the edge of Central Park. The walk takes place throughout the southeastern quadrant of the park, starting near Artists' Gate and ending near Bow Bridge. Accompanying the audio are five photographs (three of which depict an unnamed woman with long dark hair) and a map. Genre-wise, the piece explores flâneur-detective tropes with psychogeographical elements. Thematically, it draws on a variety of overlapping narratives and allusions, including, of course, oblique references to Ophelia—but there is also the JFK assassination, opera intermezzos, monologues from passers-by on the street, the sound of rain and birds, conversations between mothers and children at the zoo, quotations from Charles Baudelaire's poetry, frequent references to the mysterious woman with black hair, and excerpts from the testimony of an enslaved man named Harry Thomas—among many other subtle interjections.

Theatre and sound studies scholar Rosemary Klich identifies multiple overlapping trends in immersive theatre, audio theatre, headphone theatre, ambulatory arts practices, and so-called "secret" theatre (366). She writes that "recent headphone theatre productions use binaural and surround sound techniques to embrace an aesthetic of digital simulation" (366). This simulation is largely a function of the headphones themselves:

> The psychoacoustics of headphones produce a vivid imagining of one's own 'headspace.' As Charles Stankievech writes in "From Stethoscopes to Headphones," his article tracing the trajectory of listening, "[a] modern technological prosthetic, headphones are quite literally a bracketing of the world for a precise analysis of sound, allowing for a focused investigation into a 'phenomenology of interiority.'" Headphones produce an effect that acoustic engineers call 'in-head' acoustic imaging, which involves the perception of a space not out there in the world but inside one's own head: we become keenly aware of the 'space between the ears.' (375)

The present analysis is nothing if not a focused investigation into interiority. Cardiff's walk uses specific techniques to heighten the work's sense of "withinness"—binaural recordings, for example. Binaural audio is recorded using a dummy head with in-ear microphones to recreate the three-dimensional space of the recording, making for highly nuanced and life-like spatialization. Moreover, the environmental sounds beyond the headphones only further reinforce the interiority experienced within them (not as a rule, but as an occasional and sometimes incidental effect). In this section, I survey Cardiff's sonic representations of interiority and the simulatory mechanics that give form to her staging of Ophelian madness.

Close Listening: *Her Long Black Hair*

To orient ourselves, perhaps it would be useful to respond to some of the existing discourse around this production and particularly some of the stronger claims that have been made about it. While Laura Dorwart suggests that it is "irrelevant" whether Cardiff belongs to a "particular category of difference" such as the mad movement or the disability community, but as I will suggest, this often means that an artist has lesser stakes in the representational politics that directly impact the communities being addressed. In Dorwart's estimation, it is sufficient that Cardiff constructs "a site of imagination" where "neurologically atypical" people can see or hear themselves represented; however, I would argue that the quality of this representation is paramount. Dorwart suggests that in the audio walk "neurologically atypical individuals can imagine themselves into a community (at least of two) where non-normative and even 'deviant' ways of thinking are privileged, woven into the aesthetic, and made beautiful" (14). Within the first minute of the walk, however, a line spoken by the narrator suggests precisely the opposite: "it is loud here, isn't it? When you're in a city like New York, you have to think of all the sounds like they're a symphony, otherwise you go a bit crazy" (Cardiff, "Track 1" 00:00:25). Here, the narrator literally compels the listener to follow a normative script of listening, or risk going insane, characterizing craziness as an antithetical experience. It is telling, too, that Cardiff chooses the symphony as a perceptual regime, with its particular historical conventions and codes of conduct. With this directive to listen symphonically, I, as a listener, fail to detect space for deviant ways of thinking. In fact, Cardiff's framing of the work as a coping strategy, a way of organizing sonic information into a more tolerable and less "crazy" form, seems to oppose the mad politics of listening. Dorwart concedes that, with this line, Cardiff offers up "both an antidote to and representation of madness" (4). But the expression nullifies itself if one tries to make it stand for both things: 'you have to think mad, otherwise you go a bit crazy.' That Cardiff stigmatizes craziness in the first few seconds of the audio walk does not make a strong case for the work's community-building potential or for the relevance of her place within the mad pride movement.

According to Dorwart, "Cardiff asks us to walk that self-same borderline that mirrors the cliff's edge between the normalized definition of 'sanity' and chaos, or psychosis" (3). Echoing other claims we have encountered about mind-melding and overcoming an intersubjective divide, the author makes a metaphorical leap from putting prerecorded "voices in our heads" to a psychiatric diagnosis and likens this to "shared experience" (3). By contrast, I am doubtful as to whether *HLBH* demonstrates "a radical mental health politic," and I am especially wary of the "or" between chaos and psychosis (4). Although it would not be a stretch to call the audio walk chaotic, it would be inappropriate—and simply inaccurate—to liken the immersive experience to psychosis. More thought could be put into this sentiment, in terms of the image of a cliff's edge separating elevated sanity from fallen insanity, but this would be to get away from the primary focus of this section. To reorient us towards that focus: how does Cardiff represent Ophelian madness through sound, and in what ways does her approach converge and diverge from Mitchell's? To fall off the so-called cliff's edge would presumably be to get "lost" in these sounds, in their passing for "the real." As the art critic Sky Goodden puts it: "The threat of losing ourselves—whether in ourselves or to [Cardiff's voice]—is a simulated madness" (31). We should perhaps listen to a few of these sounds more closely to see where this "threat" of losing oneself in simulated madness resides, and what representational dynamics underlie Cardiff's simulatory soundscape.

Directly following this line, Cardiff opens up a floodgate of city sounds, like a municipal orchestra tuning up before a concert. Suggestively, the word "crazy" is followed by a dense overlapping of emergency sirens, crossing-guard whistles, and someone laying in on a car horn, which crossfades into an accordion playing the exact same note (Cardiff, "Track 1" 00:00:32). The verisimilitude of these overlappings—the notion that they were all captured in a single take rather than being multi-tracked in a computer after the fact—is highly doubtful. In a physical context, these layers would no doubt stack even further with additional sirens, unpredictable fanfares, and other noisy interjections from the outside world. Here in the forensic listening conditions of my room, the constructedness of Cardiff's Central Park is clear-cut, and indeed the cuts are quite literally clearer. The clip-clopping of horses distinctively fades in volume rather than gaining audible distance. In Schaub's walk book, Cardiff plainly describes the intended effect of these forced transitions: "We had to go to the Rambles, the forest-like part of the park, to find an area to do quiet footsteps without the traffic noise. Then we will edit them into the first section, which is supposed to give you a sense of 'nature' when you come down the stairs" (41). In this sense, the artist's process is at odds with the narrator's directive, since she seeks to capture clean recordings and enact clean breaks between sanitized nature and crazy-making culture. Recall that Harpin described Mitchell's directorial practice as one that "re-enacts orthodox psychiatry's tidying away of life's mess" and one might say something similar about Cardiff's approach to field recording (206). That being said, it is not as though *HLBH* is as straightforward as a conventional walking tour. Based on her own experience of the walk's pleasant disorientations, Dorwart speculates that "what might have been experienced by a neurotypical individual as disturbing, chaotic, alienating, or devoid of meaning was far more comprehensible, palatable, and relatable than a guided tour or meditation that resists flights of fancy or even hallucination and hauntings" (13). And yet the walk's overall success suggests a widespread appeal on par with other public immersive experiences. By contrast, Sara Ivry at *The New York Times* says that "for many participants it will be, above all, an entertainment, accompanied by headsets" (par. 4). Whether it is a tidy entertainment or a hallucinatory frolic, the piece stages madness through specific auditory techniques and it is not enough to say one way or the other without unpacking the devices at play.

One of Cardiff's notable strategies for hallucinatory sound design, for example, is the proximal staggering of voices near and far—from sounds placed at such a distance that certain snippets are hard to discern, to sounds placed with such an immediate presence that it is no wonder they feel almost brain-generated to some listeners. Take, for instance, the moment when a chorus of "hellos" erupt from a scatter plot of locations relative to Cardiff's dummy head microphones (Cardiff, "Track 1" 00:07:20), versus the moment when Cardiff's partner George speaks over top of the narrator in a soft ASMR voice, as though his mouth were whispering just millimetres away from one's head—and yet his voice seems de-spatialized, as though recorded in a soundproof room and not within the Central Park milieu. In theatre and sound scholar Ross Brown's words, such moments have "the flâneuristic, theatrical effect of spacing and re-spacing, as the aural body perpetually recalibrates itself according to head-sound superimposed on the estranged external environment" (74). With reference to Cardiff's audio walks, Ross describes "how the narrative component of the mobile headphone dispositive mimics the way the voice in one's head tells us a story about the surrounding world" (73). Here, George's voice mimics a common aesthetic in simulations of voice hearing wherein sounds from disparate contexts produce disorienting crosstalk. Adding to this fictional recreation of mad subjectivity, the narrator encourages paranoia: “I keep thinking I hear someone behind us, but we can’t look back. It is one of the rules today. He wasn’t supposed to but he did” (Cardiff, “Track 1” 00:04:35). No doubt rooted in moments such as this one, there is a strong precedent among Cardiff’s critics to discuss her work in pathological terms. In *The Walk Book*, for example, Schaub asks “Who or what is talking to us in Cardiff’s walks?” and wonders if it might be the voice of the repressed—to which she responds: “Psychotics suffering from paranoia often report hearing ‘voices’ that plague them by issuing commands or mocking them” (167). In a similar vein, but with slightly less diagnostic baggage from clinical psychiatry, Dorwart suggests that Cardiff “mirrors the mental acrobatics often experienced by the neurologically atypical (whether temporarily or as a result of longer-term mental illness) mind” (2). There are a few problems with this claim, not least of all the fact that mental illness (if we want to call it that) comes in many shapes and sizes of acrobat. And who can say what is typical of the atypical?

At one point in the walk, two loud gunshots erupt and the narrator says, “Do you hear that? They’re shooting the scavengers, the wild goats and pigs” (Cardiff, “Track 2” 00:02:55). Theatre and film scholar Marla Carlson calls this a moment of “dangerous strangeness” wherein Cardiff collapses past, present, and future into a mini-narrative (403). While it is true that pigs once roamed Manhattan and ate garbage in the streets, the narrator describes these events in the present tense, which adds an element of fantasy to the walk for listeners unfamiliar with the historicity of these events. The gunshots also call to mind negative and racist perceptions of neighbourhood crime in New York’s urban centres, while reframing such distorted and stereotypical expectations through surreal auditory imagery that exceeds so-called rational evaluation.

In another segment, Cardiff inserts audio from a CNN newscast about a bystander’s reaction to the JFK assassination. In both cases, we are presented with bullets reverberating throughout history and coming to occupy the same space, just as the narrator’s experience overlaps with the listener’s. Are these images, I wonder, truly mirror-like representations of a neurologically atypical mind? Do all atypical minds hear gunshots on a sunny afternoon in Central Park? Does one think in crossfades and voiceovers? What I am trying to suggest is that these are specific formal strategies for representing a theory of mind.

Art historian Ruth Bretherick interprets *HLBH* as a statement on women's walking and the dangers encountered therein, and she too identifies a streak of paranoia within the narrator's digressions—a perceptual schema that Cardiff displaces onto the listener (436). Bretherick argues that the walk's headphone component allows the participant to share the consciousness of the narrator by mapping the narrator's body and voice onto the participant, as a result of which "the artist's voice seems to become one's own, as she observes the surroundings, uttering thoughts that are already semi-present in one's own mind" (443). In this case, it is significant that this other person, the narrator, is coded as mad, paranoid, and hysterical. Bretherick goes on to suggest that "Cardiff's fragmented, partial, and inconclusive narratives might echo the disjointed and multilingual expressions of the hysteric" as an act of reappropriation (437). She acknowledges, however, that reappropriating the "phonic traits of the hysteric" presents an issue insofar as it establishes "the female subject as always mad and forever disenfranchised" (437). Seeing this as an impasse to a satisfactory feminist analysis, Bretherick centres her analysis instead around Cardiff's denial of visual gratification, dismantling of the male gaze, and subversion of the ideology of woman-as-body.

Perhaps the very spectrality of Cardiff's women, their absent presence in this audio walk, accounts for the gradual fading of Ophelia from the centre of my analysis. And maybe this invisibility is genuinely productive in the sense that it shores up the character from close reading—from becoming a set of signs and symbols to dismantle. Or maybe to "release woman from the space of the visual," as Bretherick puts it, is to enact another fraught reappropriation by once again rendering the character invisible (443). According to Dorwart, this production's Ophelia is "fundamentally unknowable and inaccessible," but it is this very unknowability that offers "one possible 'escape' for the perpetually trapped" character (8). We have seen in Mitchell's production, however, that silence cuts both ways. Recall Escolme's position on Ophelia's perpetual reconfinement: she argues that the Victorians likewise rendered the character immaterial to "save her from horrid theatrical sacrifice" (176). No doubt Mitchell's forensic aesthetics are in part a response to this idea that Ophelia is "far too soft" to "fall and bleed" (176). By comparison, Cardiff's aesthetics live predominantly on the non-forensic surface, in snippets of overheard dialogue and conversations without beginning or end.

If it is true, as Escolme says, that "ideas about insanity produce Ophelia" at the same time as "Ophelia produces ideas about insanity" then we should listen more closely to those moments when Cardiff's narrator passes by random strangers who mutter to themselves in recognizably mad inflections. At one point, she passes a man who says "No respect, do not get no respect, no no no no" (Cardiff, "Track 1" 00:08:08) and then, seconds later, she passes a woman who says "the colour yellow makes him depressed and he won't eat any food that's yellow and four yellow cars in a row means a very bad day" (Cardiff, "Track 1" 00:08:30). This overheard speech has an archetypal if not stereotypical quality, in that it presents a highly legible if not symbolic madness—in the first case, someone talking to himself, and in the second case, an example of magical thinking. If not forensic, this mode of listening—one of overhearing or eavesdropping—could be called voyeuristic (or auralistic, for lack of a better term). How is madness formally constructed here, one might ask, and how does this construction produce Ophelia? According to Bree Hadley: "The fact that these personae are produced by spectators not by biology is, for disability scholars, activists and artists, demonstrated by the plethora of imagery spectators and societies have attached to their bodies over time," which is also true of auditory representations (4). This dynamic is fundamentally absent, if not occluded, from many discussions around simulated madness, which presume that mad auralities are a concrete phenomenon that can be reproduced, and not co-constructions of the artist and listener.

One further consideration is that, in these moments, madness is not a shared headphone experience, but exists figuratively *over there* among strangers, whose mad voices clash with Cardiff's rational and authoritative narrator, who issues verbal commands like only someone in command of their faculties would (or so to speak). These snippets of overheard speech, then, are not just representations of mad vocality; rather, stereotypical mad utterances orient us, as listeners, towards stereotypical listening.

Conclusion

In a foundational study of objectival representations of mental illness, Ellen W. Kaplan surveys the formal means by which artists render the psyche on stage, using theatrical space to mirror thoughts. A messy room might be chosen to convey disordered thinking, for example (78). These representations are never neutral, however, and in fact they are often troublesome. The danger—and the irony—of cementing something like a "theatre of psychosis," for example, is that it threatens to formalize the very thing it suggests is marked by formal dissolution. As Kaplan puts it, "the experience of mental illness cannot be so much explained as depicted, embodied in form, structure, object as metaphor. Even these strategies are partial, calls from the edge" (88). As such, I write towards qualifying, nuancing, and de-absolutizing these strategies, as well as troubling the claims that are made about them.

Too often, the experience of intersubjectivity is rendered in absolute terms, as if it were a form of telepathy, and these are precisely the kinds of claims that warrant reevaluation. Indeed, the concept of intersubjective listening has considerable representational and ethical stakes: how do we—without the capacity for direct knowledge of others—formally imagine ourselves in their point of audition? Moreover, what are the consequences of different forms of imaginative engagement? For me, the two works under comparison in this chapter offer a way to investigate these questions by way of contrast; a comparative analysis provides an opportunity to highlight different modes of perception and mediation, different ways of externalizing and representing thought, and different aesthetics of acoustic interiority.

Writing about Elizabethan literature, Drew Daniel describes intersubjectivity as "tantalizingly partial, incomplete yet undeniable" (90). According to him, the theoretical function of Hamlet's asides, for example, is to press the audience "asymptotically closer to a representation of instantaneous thought, of an inner flicker of consciousness rather than a practiced performance of speech" (141). Formally, the aside creates a sense of dramatic access, a mind open to spectators but closed to other characters. Shuffling between insides, outsides, and asides, Daniel theorizes melancholy as an assemblage, something existing in excess of the individual, in "a network of dynamic, interpretive relationships between persons, bodies, texts, spaces, structures, and things" (iv). In a non-subjective framework like this one, so-called telepathic access is rendered moot. There is no "there" there, as Daniel reminds us, quoting Gertrude Stein. In other words, neither melancholy nor madness is seated exclusively in the mind but in a complex array of interrelations and spaces of encounter. In a basic sense, then, the promise of acoustic "interiority" is a false one, because mad aurality exceeds pure interiority. This idea is reflected in the medical framework of "mental" illness, which situates madness exclusively within minds, at the expense of ignoring its social constructedness (in whole or in part, depending on who you ask). Contrast this with Mitchell's approach in *OZ*, where madness is largely figured as a mental state. According to Harpin, even though the play attempts to show "the asphyxiating patriarchal conditions that produce women's despair," its portrayal of madness as an "internal catastrophe" is nevertheless politically regressive (197).

Sonic representations of mad auralities trigger a specific kind of interpretive dynamic, calling attention to epistemological limits. Indeed, Daniel suggests that such representations activate the boundary between sympathy and scepticism (3). I posit *mad listening* as a means of keeping this tension alive—that of surface and depth, interior access and exterior opacity, signification, and non-representation. Mad listening, in other words, is an orientation, a way of making sense of the gap between identification and estrangement. Moreover, it is a technique for bearing witness to an area of critical tension. In this chapter, I have argued for more nuance, and fewer absolutes, in the hypothesizing of shared auralities. Between Dorwart's argument that Cardiff makes it compulsory to think madly, and Montironi's argument that Mitchell compels listeners to share Ophelia's mad earpoint, one of the more common assumptions around shared auralities would appear to be the selling-out of close formal analysis for easy leaps to empathic experience.

The underdetermined aspects of mad listening stand in bold contrast to the overdetermined aspects of what I might call *factitious* listening. By contrast, the factitious listener takes realism, simulation, and analogical fixity for granted, trying on madness as though it were a pair of headphones. The term "factitious" refers to a diagnosed and so-called disordered form of malingering, but I use it in the vernacular sense of an affective contrivance. My aim is not to police the boundaries between "real" and "fake" madness, however. As disability studies scholar Ellen Samuels reminds us, "what we mean by 'fake disability' will always be blurry, contingent, and incomplete" because disability inherently confounds attempts at classification (71). Nonetheless, we need nuanced language to describe particular orientations towards madness and the ways in which it is consumed and created. Factitious listening goes with the grain of authorial intent and operates within what sound studies scholar Brian Kane calls *onto-aesthetics*, "a belief that works of art can disclose their ontology" outside of cultural context (2). During encounters with staged madness, auditors are often invited to experience what it is like to be mad, put in relation to mad *beingness*—quite often along diagnostic lines. Though the mad-sane binary is problematic—and I do not mean to recreate it by proposing a mad/factitious split—it is necessary to prioritize lived experience over metaphor. Mad and factitious listening do not represent a binary so much as they represent two of many possible interpretive strategies. I have plucked these terms from their respective corners for the same reason that I have chosen these two contrasting case studies; that is, to explicate different modes of representation and interpretation.

Rather than policing the boundaries of madness, we ought to sketch these boundaries with as much detail as possible. Take Megan Ratner's review of *HLBH*, for example, in which the author suggests that "Cardiff's voice seems to emanate from within your head rather than from outside your ears, a level of intimacy both beguiling and invasive" (par. 1). It is assertions such as this one that prompted the present examination, and which open up a problem space for further analysis. What mechanisms are behind the *seeming*? What material conditions are behind the *emanation*? What props up such fantasies of intersubjectivity? What is acoustic interiority made up of? What is the relationship between proximity and reality, intimacy and truth? What must we bracket to be beguiled, and what must we accept to be entrained? In the next chapter, I recontextualize these questions by addressing additional intersections, particularly around the convergence of mad auralities and racialized sound.

Notes

1. Consider, for example, Ruth Breckerick's "The Urge to Disappear: Janet Cardiff's Audio Walks in London and New York" (2021), or Amy Spencer's "Literary Thresholds: Exploring the Edges of Ambient Literature" (2018).
2. The Foley sounds are provided by Glyn Pritchard (Polonius), Ulrich Hoppe (Laertes), and Renato Schuch (Hamlet), who play double roles in this regard. They produce traditional Foley footsteps and door slams, as well as other offstage sound effects (distant voices, etc.).
3. My analysis of Mitchell's performance references and relies exclusively on a video copy provided by the Schaubühne theatre: such are the exigencies of writing in the time of a pandemic. Without a doubt, my experience of the work is highly detached as a result,

but I hope to avoid any significant interpretive lapses by focusing primarily on sound.

4. In short, Harpin argues that Mitchell's work "repeatedly sustains cultural narratives of female madness as ultimately, and always, personal, catastrophic affliction," and does so through a forensic or diagnostic lens (196–197). By contrast, Montironi argues that by "sharing Ophelia's acoustic world, spectators can fully tune into the character and better understand her subjugation, as well as the violence perpetrated against her by patriarchal society" (133).
5. Here, I echo Montironi's usage of "earpoint," though I prefer the term "point of audition" so as to deemphasize the primacy of the ear as an organ of listening. In *Theater of the Mind Imagination, Aesthetics, and American Radio Drama* (2012), media studies scholar Neil Verma also proposes the term "audioposition" to emphasize the fact that this positioning is a representational gesture, i.e., not just a noun but also a verb.

CHAPTER 4

Staging Medicine and Sounding Madness in Suvendrini Lena's *Here Are the Fragments*

Here are the Fragments (2019) is an immersive theatre installation, created by Suvendrini Lena, and co-directed by Leah Cherniak and Mumbi Tindyebwa Otu. Through a combination of scripted scenes, interactive elements, and spatial dramaturgy, the play explores the intersection of racism and mental health, inspired by Frantz Fanon's writings. According to Ian Baucom, Fanon was not just a "visual anatomist of imperialism" but also a theorist of sound who continues "to teach us about the audible" (16). Baucom suggests that Fanonian listening locates radical solidarity in a "collective dissent of interpretation" (35) rather than notions of "being alike" or "hearing alike" (29). Such dissent might include attending to "gaps in the record, in the vacant place where something, perhaps, should have been but was not" (47). It is in moments of "fragmentation and incompleteness," says Baucom, that a soundscape "speaks its invitation to an audience for whom the real task of reconstruction will then begin" (47). The production in question makes just such an invitation.

Here are the Fragments draws its title from Frantz Fanon's *Black Skin, White Masks* (1967) in which he wrote "the Other fixes me with his gaze, his gestures and attitude, the same way you fix a preparation with a dye. I lose my temper, demand an explanation…Nothing doing. I explode. Here are the fragments put together by another me" (89). Here, Fanon describes the effect of the white colonial gaze as one of fragmentation.

M. Tomkinson, *Sound and Sense in Contemporary Theatre*,
https://doi.org/10.1007/978-3-031-78034-9_4

After being hailed with a racial epithet, the author experiences a splitting of his identity between his sense of self-identity and his "being for others" (89). This splitting is referenced in the title of the play and further reflected in the production's wider themes, as well as its narrative shards.

For context, since this play is less well-known than the others I have discussed so far: this installation ran from November 19th to December 1st of 2019 at The Theatre Centre in Tkaronto (Toronto), which is situated on unceded Anishnaabe, Huron-Wendat, and Haudenosaunee territory. It was co-produced by The ECT Collective, a not-for-profit theatre company based in St. Catharines. The playwright, Suvendrini Lena, teaches psychiatry at the University of Toronto and is also a staff neurologist at The Centre for Addiction and Mental Health (CAMH). Five years before the premiere of this play, Lena taught a seminar, in collaboration with the playwright Colleen Murphy, called "Staging Medicine," the focus of which was to "unsettle our ideas of disease and healing" (Peterkin par. 1). The writeup for this seminar tells participants that they will "enter directly into the world of psychosis, suicide, cancer, and dementia for example—in order to see and understand these states freshly and deeply" (par. 2). To similar ends, the play's promotional material presents the following prompt to audiences: "Within our immersive design (a fabric of sound, video, and live actors) lean in close to the possibilities of perceptual experience" ("Residency" par. 2). This notion of "leaning in close" to the experience of voice hearing is echoed in a number of reviews. For example, Ilana Lucas suggests that the play provides "a chance to slip under a different skin and into a different mind, and to feel the Other in yourself" (par. 13).[1]

Representing this sense of difference and otherness is Dr. Frantz Chauvet (Allan Louis), the play's Black protagonist, who not only treats so-called schizophrenia as a psychiatrist but comes to hear voices himself. One of Dr. Chauvet's voices belongs to the revolutionary psychiatrist and philosopher Frantz Fanon, whose personal library has been recreated in the set. Audiences can freely access this library as they wander through the performance space. The aforementioned reviewer, Lucas, describes the set as a series of "jewel-box rooms," including an office, a series of cubicles, a hospital bed, open spaces where headphones dangle from the ceiling, a lecture space, a projection wall representing a street corner, a forest scene, and more (par. 10). In her pre-show speech, Lena invites audience members to interact with whatever grabs their attention: "you can touch objects, you can turn on tape recorders, you can listen to headphones, you can speak into microphones, you can lean into radios, you can stand close to the actors: it is an intimate experience" ("Draft One" 00:01:40–00:02:00).

As is perhaps to be expected with immersive theatre, some audience members are comfortable in an information-heavy space, whereas other attendees have described the open-mindedness of the production as an "overwhelming bombardment of sensory stimuli" (Dugalin n.pag). Of the dozen or so reviews that exist online, most conclude that this sensory bombardment is intended to replicate the sensory experience of voice hearing. Indeed, to the point of biological determinism, Lucas suggests that the production's set design, with its "floor-to-ceiling wires," evokes "the electrical impulses of the brain that dictate who we are and what we do" (par. 11). Altogether, then, one can detect a common and familiar appeal to the intersubjective, to the mechanisms by which one imagines oneself into another's headspace; meanwhile, it is this very headspace that people tend to imagine, by default, as the locus of "mental" illness.

This chapter attends to many of the action verbs quoted above: to *enter directly* into the world of psychosis, to *lean in* to another's perception, to *slip under* another's skin and be immersed in their head, as if walking around in it, touching objects and turning on tape recorders. It is worth noting, however, that once again I have experienced this production strictly through video documentation, and as a result, there has been no occasion for sensory bombardment of the sort described above. Yet, it bears repeating that if there is any upside to experiential distance here, perhaps it prevents one from being enchanted by the exaggerated promises and affective charges of immersion. Nevertheless, it would be futile to argue whether immersion is effective or ineffective from the position of a non-participant. Rather, the following analysis is more specifically concerned with the aesthetics and politics of simulation, as expressed in Lena's sonic representations of madness.

Apropos of sound, *Fragments* has been described as a "hauntingly resonant" play: in context, Lisa McKoewn writes that "some scenes are hauntingly resonant illustrations of Chauvet's mental unravelling" (par. 7). To what extent, I wonder, can the concept of resonance help clarify the play's social reverberations? On one side, the political paradigm of "resonance" might move beyond the realms of sanism by way of challenging the standard dynamic of signification and interpretation. As Jean-Luc Nancy puts it, resonance might be thought of as "beyond-sense or sense that goes beyond signification" (31). Yet, by trying to move beyond signification, one might miss the nuances of representation, including the ways that certain misleading assumptions about madness are inscribed in sound. Questions around resonance are bound up with the problematics of simulation. According to the composer and sound studies theorist Suzanne Thorpe, "while we make our way through our days, we may notice that, as we listen to external sounds, we also hear those same sounds sonified internally" (82). Thorpe is cautious of "sameness," however: she proceeds from the understanding that resonance can be both a "referent for hegemonic normativity" (e.g., audism) and also a medium for intersubjectivity, entanglement, and relational truth (86).

In his review of the play, Istvan Dugalin writes that the central theme of *Fragments*—"the core that resonates through it all"—is Dr. Chauvet's maddening experience of institutional racism (par. 7). This chapter asks how we might parse these reverberations. Where do they emerge from? What are they made of? With whom do they resonate, and how? Mad studies scholar La Marr Jurelle Bruce reminds us that the same representation can carry both "radical resonance and capitulation to stereotype" (223). Accounting for this ambivalence, I approach *Fragments* with close attention to resonant stereotypes and stereotypical resonances. My own position on resonance is highly ambivalent in this regard, to the extent that this concept can operate as both a powerful unifier and a thought-terminating cliché.[2] In the same vein, Will Schrimshaw argues that the "logic of interiority," insofar as it represents the guiding ideology of immersion, "diminishes capacity for thinking beyond the immediacy of human experience, collapsing differentiation through the assertion of an affective homogeneity positing mystical unification" (*Immanence* 2). Following Schrimshaw, I treat these logics of mystical resonance and interiority as planes of immanence, while attending to the ways in which such concepts are aestheticized. In other words, focusing on "methods of representation and formalization can present exit strategies" from transcendental claims about intersubjective access (186). "A critical immersive practice," according to Schrimshaw, "requires acts of distanciation" and "entails immersion without aesthetic immediacy or sufficiency, without the conflation of image or sensorial event and reality" (193). In terms of this case study, this means taking a critical perspective on aural simulations of madness.

Though I have expressed wariness about the misapplications of resonance, my critical approach is nonetheless partly inspired by the Stó:lō sound studies scholar Dylan Robinson's notion of "resonant theory," a form of critical-affective writing that tries to capture and convey echoes of sensory experience by moving in tandem with a work of art, as opposed to forms of structural analysis that enact epistemic and material violence against other subjectivities (15). According to Robinson, one goal of performative writing in a sound studies context is to "expose normative listening practices" by identifying the writer's positionality (81). As such, it is important to note that I am engaging with this material as a white settler-scholar, and there is no doubt that Lena's play conveys knowledge beyond my own experience, critical prerogative, and authority to represent. Accordingly, I aim to expose my listening biases by emphasizing this study's limited and subjective framing—a process of acknowledging all that falls outside my range of hearing, and all that succeeds or fails to resonate for me personally. The close analysis that follows therefore travels alongside the performance footage in real time, describing the play's formal frameworks without trying to dismantle them. Though this chapter remains beholden to conventional scholarly criticism in terms of querying representational issues, I hope to employ Bruce's notion of critical ambivalence in order to "entertain some level of deliberate opacity," as Robinson puts it (102). Ultimately, I aim to formulate open-ended questions rather than reductive conclusions and to apply a filter to those frequencies which resonate most strongly with me.

Close Listening: *Here Are the Fragments*

Turning to the video documentation, housed on Vimeo, I note that the show begins with Lena delivering a land acknowledgement. She recognizes the Indigenous territory on which this performance takes place, and also states that this work pays tribute to "the ancestors of those of African origin and descent" ("Draft One" 00:01:05–00:01:10). She continues, adding: "We also acknowledge that this building stands on the grounds of the former provincial Asylum for the Insane, as it was called, until the middle of the last century" ("Draft One" 00:01:10–00:01:22). After this, the opening remarks turn to the specifics of the immersive experience that audience members are about to have. Perhaps it is because I do not live here in this city, and do not traverse these grounds every day—or perhaps this information was communicated in some other way off-screen, perhaps embedded in a playbill or some other paratext—but I sense a heavy lacuna here in acknowledging the performance site, yet passing over the asylum's institutional legacy. Moreover, the phrase "middle of the last century" lingers in my mind, and I wonder if this is meant to signify an endpoint. What has since transpired on those grounds between then and now, and how does that institution's legacy continue under the new address of 1001 Queen Street West, and the new title of the Centre for Addiction and Mental Health? Moreover, how can such histories resonate with us unless they are addressed directly, struck like a bell?

Continuing with her opening remarks, Lena invites audience members to actively immerse themselves by standing near actors, picking up objects, and putting on headphones. According to Natalie Alvarez, such moments of invitation always contain implicit, if not explicit, imperatives. "It might seem trite to assert that the immersive simulation is never merely an experienced event: it is overcoded in advance by its ideological and pedagogical imperatives and there is, typically, a debriefing, a recounting that allows these objectives to become sedimented" (12). As I have shown throughout the preceding chapters, madness simulations tend to be encoded with the combined imperative to learn and empathize by means of proximity. Referring to Sara Ahmed's work, Alvarez suggests that "there is a danger [...] in 'assuming proximity or distance as the basis of an ethics'" (99). Accordingly, throughout this chapter, I question the role of immersion in allegedly bringing audiences closer to understanding mad aural experiences.

At the three-minute mark, as the show's attendees are shown walking up a stairwell and into the performance space, a narrator's voice erupts from the right side of my headphones: "Have you ever felt that someone or something was trying to communicate directly with you, by sending special signals or signs, perhaps through a radio or television or computer or a phone?" ("Draft One" 00:03:00–00:03:30). Soon after this voice fades out, Dr. Chauvet enters and screens the audience for so-called mental illness, as a psychiatrist would, using similar questions: "Have you ever heard voices, I mean voices that other people can't hear?" ("Draft One" 00:04:30–00:04:40). My answer to both of these questions is "no," and yet the format of the questions feels familiar, since I myself have been screened on a number of occasions, by medical professionals wielding intake forms headlined by cryptic combinations of numbers and acronyms. Supposing that other audience members may have answered "yes" to these questions, I can only imagine that such an immersive scenario could potentially be retraumatizing. This incongruity underscores a peculiar feature of immersive mental health plays, which is that the simulation does not necessarily imagine someone with lived experience (the *simulated*) as a primary audience member.

Nevertheless, we are made to imagine, if only for the duration of the performance, that we inhabit their reality. Dr. Chauvet speaks of words that are "somehow inserted into your head, directly or indirectly," as if to call attention to the set of headphones I am wearing, through which the actor's voice is transmitted into my ears, and into my head ("Draft One" 00:04:45–00:04:50). From the outset, voice hearing is framed in a highly medicalized fashion, with an overt emphasis on the brain: behind the actor, for example, the walls of the performance space are adorned with media cables resembling dendrites, along with projections of actual dendrite structures, shown pulsing with neural activity. One should take the aforementioned course title, "Staging Medicine" at face value in this case.

Yet, the play shows a keen awareness of medical authority and the ways in which it is wielded and withheld. Indeed, Dr. Chauvet's transition from doctor to patient arrives suddenly, as he is stripped of authority in the span of a costume change. No sooner does he finish screening the audience than his lab coat is forcibly removed, and he is helped into a cardigan and toque. At this point, the show's soundscape, designed by Nick Murray, also undergoes a dramatic change. The room is now awash with subtle clicks, piercing tones, and sullen piano chords. Adding to this cacophony with his voice, Dr. Chauvet sits down at a table, repetitively uttering a single syllable to himself, which sounds variously like "tuh" or "tap" or "took" ("Draft One" 00:07:45–00:08:00). Meanwhile, his twenty-four-year-old son Eduard (Kwaku Adu-Poku), from whom he has been estranged for fifteen years, approaches the table and offers him a home-cooked meal. It turns out, however, that this doctor, once in charge of others, has had his own bodily autonomy revoked, and is now forbidden from eating with cutlery.

It is here that Lena introduces the play's main intertext, Fanon's *Black Skin, White Masks*, from which Eduard reads an underlined passage to his father: "the Other fixes me with his gaze, his gestures and attitude, the same way you fix a preparation with a dye. I lose my temper, demand an explanation…Nothing doing. I explode. Here are the fragments put together by another me" (89). Though Fanon writes explicitly about the white gaze—of ocularcentrism, epidermalization, and visual body-schemas—this scene conveys similar issues, related to the objectification of Blackness and madness, through sound.

Despite the similarities, however, there is some representational dissonance to be accounted for here. On one side, Dr. Chauvet is reduced to a medical archetype that reflects the pathological profile of so-called schizophrenia, as officially diagnosed in the play, and as suggested by the emphasis on his most alienating symptom—namely, his "disorganized speech." In this regard, the play itself objectifies him, making him an "object among other objects" in Fanon's sense (89). At the same time, Dr. Chauvet's mad vocality could be understood as a "resonant crack," which La Marr Jurelle Bruce defines as a moment in which "the voice cracks, breaks, snaps, and is nevertheless transmitted to audiences in its riven condition" (156). According to Bruce, such cracked resonances can expose the fissures within ideologies of systemic oppression. If Black protest songs, as per Bruce, can be "wordless exclamations of fury at racial injustice," then Dr. Chauvet's wordless utterances might be heard and understood in similar terms (156). That is to say: his mad vocalizations are a valid response to a highly oppressive environment, and consequently the play's emphasis on Dr. Chauvet's symptomatology is not meant to stereotype him as a so-called schizophrenic, but to index injustice—the removal of his right and authority to speak.

Following Bruce, I approach this scene with critical ambivalence, noting that two different interpretations are possible and that we may "object to its problematic contents even as we endorse its progressive potential" (211). To this end, we should be cautious with resonant critiques, in case we are moved for the wrong reasons. In *Fragments*, we find both complex criticism and antimad material, both "radical resonance and capitulation to stereotype" (223). Lena's inclination towards a more scientific interpretation of voice hearing exposes another interpretive double-bind with which we might struggle as listeners, since *Fragments* challenges systemic injustice from within an institutional and, even more explicitly, medical framework. I acknowledge, however, that such ambivalence may indeed be easier to practice from where I am sitting, at a distance.

In the following scene, Dr. Chauvet is once again helped into his lab coat as the heavy gears of a machine begin audibly to turn. Next, the room darkens, and a swarm of whispers emerges overhead. Certain plosive phrases stand out from the dense swirl of sound, including expressions one might expect to hear in popular representations of madness. One voice, for example, speaks of "devils put there to torture me," before being cut off by the noise of radio interference ("Draft One"

00:13:10–00:13:25). Exiting the waiting room, audience members now spill through a large set of doors into the open interactive space of the theatre. In the hallway, we meet the ghost of a woman who calls herself Ether (Kyra Harper), otherwise known as Alice, who died from maltreatment and now haunts the premises. In the left ear of my headphones, Ether describes the walls on which she writes as a "schizo-palimpsest," while in my right ear, Dr. Chauvet's voice says: "A schizophrenic is a survivor of self-loss" ("Draft One" 00:14:35–00:14:42). Their overlapping voices only intensify the interpretive tension I discussed above, by putting an allegedly sane voice in one ear (that of a medical doctor providing a diagnosis), and a supposedly mad voice in the other (that of a patient speaking to herself in a songlike intonation). For me, these voices do not harmonize or resonate so much as they create a productive dissonance. In effect, this listening situation reflects particular aesthetic conventions around representing voice hearing, and yet, thinking back to Schrimshaw, we should not readily conflate sound design with lived experience.

As the camera travels to the next room, we encounter a group of audience members wearing headphones not unlike my own. I cannot be sure that we are listening to the same thing, though this may always be the case in a more abstract sense. Regardless, it is clear that these headphones play a key role in representing the sensory experience of voice hearing. Beyond representing other states of mind, headphones are sometimes discussed in terms of cultivating intersubjective resonance, and thereby sharing a mental state. Erica Fretwell, a literary sound studies scholar, discusses the telephone in a similar vein, as a vehicle for "psychical interconnection" which brings atomized subjects into "sympathetic vibration" (102). Fretwell underscores the telephone's utopian function in late nineteenth-century literature and culture—specifically, its alleged ability to facilitate "a kind of transpersonal solidarity, the porous, boundless consciousness that the utopian state requires" (102).[3]

To comparable ends, Lena uses a combination of microphones and headphones to simulate voice hearing for audience members. When some audience members speak into a free-standing microphone, the sounds they make are transmitted directly to headphones worn by other participants on the opposite side of the room. In this way, Lena's direct feed of voices, like Fretwell's telephone, provides the show with a "material infrastructure of transpersonal consciousness" (103). As I have already suggested, this infrastructure is not simply a medium for sharing in the lived experience of voice hearing; rather, it provides an embodied experience that acts as a material metaphor for the auditory symptoms associated with this diagnosis. Speaking to this formal device, Carly Maga writes the following in her review of the play: "it's a fascinating simulation of mental illness and one that's a relief to escape after 90 minutes and not have to carry within oneself every day" (par. 8). If the play carries a lasting resonance, then, such sympathetic vibrations would appear to quickly taper off, and for some people, desirably so. As can readily be seen from this example, the so-called "relief of escape" which is so fundamental to disability and madness simulations ultimately works against destigmatization. Valerie Brew-Parrish, a vocal critic of disability simulations, observes this same tendency of participants to "breathe a collective sigh of relief knowing full well that their charade will soon come to an end and their momentary disability will gratefully vanish" (2). To my mind, such gestures of recoiling signal a rejection of resonance, a turning away, and an underlining of the privilege of having agency to dip in and out of an experience.

As I return once more to the video documentation, contemplating the movement of participants as they wander from room to room, and reflecting on my mediated engagement with this space and its embodied dimensions, I cannot help but think of the historical phenomenon of asylum tourism, together with the contemporary enthusiasm for interactive productions set in fictional asylums (often staged in formerly active institutions). It is beyond the scope of this chapter to discuss this topic in-depth, but it is important to note the precedence for this particular mode of immersive theatre. According to the medical historian Janet Miron, "the practice continued at the Toronto Asylum well into the late nineteenth century, as it did at all other public asylums in Ontario" (31). Putting aside any questions as to the incentives and ramifications of this practice, I am simply struck by the inaudibility of this context, a missing fundamental of sorts in the overall spectrum of the production, which, if made to resonate more fully, might complicate participants' desire to "enter directly into the world of psychosis," and the privileged exit that is implied ("Staging Medicine" par. 2). With the context of asylum tourism in mind, such exciting assurances begin to sound more like transgressions, including the invitation to stand close to the actors as they perform the role of patients. Indeed, this historical practice often relied on a similar dynamic of watching without being seen and listening without being heard (Miron 34). Likewise, the value of such asylum visits was attached to ideals of education, sympathy, or—most unsettlingly—entertainment. How, I ask, might we experience *Fragments* differently in light of this "sadistic pastime," as Miron calls it (35)? This is not to suggest that the installation actively carries on this pastime, only that it necessarily bears this historical resonance.

As one of the next scenes starts, I come to the delayed realization that my experience of the play has been rendered linear, if still highly fragmentary: the camera cuts between noteworthy moments, rather than drifting aimlessly, as a participant might. Now, we are back with Dr. Chauvet, who, in the course of dictating his clinical notes into a hand-held tape machine, reveals to the audience that he has been mistaken for a janitor ("Draft One" 00:17:10–00:17:20). Here, the whispering continues in my right ear, except now there are three distinct voices, including that of the doctor, his son, and Ether. At times, Dr. Chauvet speaks in two voices: not only his natural voice but also an overdubbed voice, implied to be an internal dialogue. At other moments, these overdubs are louder than the voices in the room, masking the characters' live speech. One of these voices, presumably belonging to Ether, repetitively commands someone, presumably Dr. Chauvet, to "Stop talking!" ("Draft One" 00:21:45–00:21:55). Admittedly, since I myself experience repetitive intrusive thoughts, some of these sound design techniques are, for lack of a better word, triggering. For a moment, I entertain the notion of relief, prompted by the Theatre Centre website, where the following imperatives appear: "Within the installation find places of retreat from chaos. Find poetry. Find critical analysis" ("Residency Page" par. 3). You may be wondering, as I am, what the word "chaos" refers to here: perhaps the bustling audience, or the world at large that overwhelms us, or madness itself? If it indeed refers to the latter, as it must to some extent in this context, then such a slippage between madness and chaos draws our attention to one of the most common stigmas attached to so-called schizophrenia. Quoting the psychiatrist Robert Barrett on stigma, Bruce reminds us that medicalized madness is often "reduced to a negative sign," and schizophrenia in particular is frequently "co-opted to 'represent symbolically much of what has gone wrong in the modern world,' forcing voice-hearers to bear 'the responsibility of representing an alienated, fragmented, meaningless, self-absorbed society'" (15). The question for me, as a mad listener engaging with this play, is this: how can we reclaim chaos, such that it is not framed as something to be retreated from?

Far from chaotic, many of the play's thematic strands come together with relative tidiness. In an earlier scene, Eduard approaches an audience member, breaking the immersive fourth wall, and asks her to interpret a line from his father's clinical notes: "Medication is the biochemistry of loss" ("Draft One" 00:15:25–00:15:45). Later, an overdubbed voice belonging to Dr. Chauvet echoes this statement when he says: "A schizophrenic is a survivor of self-loss" ("Draft One" 00:21:45–00:21:55). If one puts the two statements together, one is led to conclude that the purpose of medication is to restore a person's sense of self, which has been lost to madness. Though one cannot disprove such a syllogism, it nonetheless announces the play's biomedical perspective on the etiology and treatment of madness. Though Lena writes from the position of a neurologist, her thoughts on healing are not so clear-cut, however. In a profile on the CAMH website, the doctor-turned-playwright says that she tries "to integrate the understanding of the brain as an organ into everything that I do," and yet she also recognizes the necessity of treating "both body and soul" (par. 17). The theatre historian Meredith Conti notes a long-sustained motif of the "dramatist-as-pathologist" on stage, meaning that any staging of a diagnostic condition takes part in constructing a particular profile of illness (7). No doubt, the playwright is aware of this phenomenon, since Dr. Chauvet remarks at one point in his clinical notes: "It is the doctor who fabricated and continues to fabricate the patient" ("Draft One" 00:26:05–00:26:11).

Within the play's profile of illness is another layer of pathological construction, largely attributable to the fictional doctors who clinically evaluate Dr. Chauvet, and who tell Eduard over the phone that his father is "not capable" ("Draft One" 00:23:30–00:23:35). By contrast, the play itself upholds Dr. Chauvet's agency, autonomy, and credibility, and in doing so makes him a foil for these other medical practitioners, embedded within the narrative. One scene in particular reveals the protagonist's desire to be better than the profession: "Here are souls, immured, visible as traces, yes—audible to me. It is for me to devise a method of electrical extraction. Yes, I choose—I choose to hear them, I choose to heal them. To read beneath the skin. I will transcend medicine" ("Draft One" 00:25:05–00:25:45). In the following scene, Dr. Chauvet makes good on his promise to heal through hearing when he sits down beside one of his patients, Alice, and refers to her by her self-given name, Ether. Furthermore, when she tells him that electricity is entering through her window, he offers to close the blinds, and finally, when Ether tries to read his mind telepathically, he confirms her suspicions ("Draft One" 00:30:00–00:32:00). In this regard, Dr. Chauvet follows a mad methodology of sorts, listening with madness rather than against it, and leaning into its resonances rather than recoiling from them. According to Bruce, to uphold a mad approach is to validate and take seriously "the purported pathology of delusion," and to find metaphysical truths within that which the rationalist deems unreasonable (43).

In some sense, the play makes this acceptance of the unreasonable easy for us, as when Dr. Chauvet stands behind a lectern delivering a speech on *Black Skin, White Masks*, and one of his voices, Frantz Fanon (Peter Bailey) appears beside him, embodied. There is no denying the truth of this so-called delusion. Fanon occasionally echoes, contradicts, interrupts, or finishes the doctor's train of thought, until the doctor is forced to engage directly with this hallucinatory presence. Fanon then confronts Dr. Chauvet, asking him whether he sees himself in the aforementioned book, as an inferiorized Black man aspiring to "gain admittance to the white world" by earning the respect of his colleagues (45). If Fanon appears to undermine Dr. Chauvet's authority here, however, it is only to set up a dramatic contrast in the following scene, wherein the doctor suddenly finds himself on the street, speaking in the familiar, frenzied cadence of a madman. From delivering speeches into a microphone situated on a platform ten feet above the ground to shouting at the top of his voice from the corridor below, Dr. Chauvet plays out a spatiolinguistic metaphor of going mad. Though both of these orientations—miked platform and unmiked street—operate on an equal plane for me as a headphone listener, one must assume that a live audience would attune to their differences with greater sensitivity. Through this spatial contrast, which borders on parody in its literal elevation of the doctor, Lena draws the audience's attention to the fictitious authority of lab coats, microphones, pedestals, and lecterns. As a result, one is left to consider the ideological and material systems that structure one's listening, particularly in relation to Blackness and madness.

Having said this, the street scene I mentioned carries an uncomfortable resonance, though it is unclear whether such discomfort is deliberate. The critical mental health researcher Sarah Redikopp suggests that "the spatialization of madness and confinement of mad people has arguably transformed from that figure 'beyond walls' to a phenomenon of hypervisibility organized through neoliberal capitalist and settler colonial organizations and distribution of poverty and precarity" (111). Moreover,

Redikopp reminds us that this dynamic is "closely informed by processes of racialization and racial cartographies" (111). In this scene, Dr. Chauvet is both hypervisible and hyperaudible, and yet goes unseen and unheard: "I ain't here. I'm in the code, encoded" he says at one point ("Draft One" 00:48:30–00:48:35). As I pay closer attention to the audience in the background, I am troubled by the choreography of this immersive spectacle: Dr. Chauvet paces up and down a corridor formed by two walls with pictures of a downtown street corner projected upon them. Here, on this simulated street corner, he alternates between mumbling quietly to himself and shouting at the top of his lungs, as a group of twenty or thirty audience members stand around him with their arms crossed, ogling and eavesdropping, real-world coffee cups in hand. Even as police sirens begin to wail in the distance, and Dr. Chauvet yells "Get your hands off me!" from some place offstage, the crowd remains unmoved ("Draft One" 00:48:50–00:49:05). Though the unsettling dramaturgy of this scene could be interpreted as a critique of the white gaze, the voyeuristic onlooker, the docile listener, the passive bystander, and the society of the spectacle more generally, it nevertheless stages an interaction that would be considered profoundly inhumane in everyday life. While immersive theatre may sometimes heighten a sense of ethical responsibility among participants, it can also give audiences implicit or explicit permission to relax their sense of social obligation, if not completely transgress it. One of the more discomfiting aspects of *Fragments*, then, is the way in which it frames voice hearing as a curio, something to be heard and observed as if from behind glass.

However, we should also notice, in the course of Dr. Chauvet's speech, further examples of the resonant crack—a break in the voice which exposes the seams in anti-Black and antimad ideology. Take the following lines, for example, which reveal the iatrogenic (i.e., medically induced) causes of Dr. Chauvet's symptoms: "I ain't sick sick sick sick sicken, lick lick lick lickin' lickin' lickin' lickin' lickin' my lips, tardive, sicken, tardive smackin', tardive dyskinesia, tardive amnesia: that is why I'm fuckin' lickin' my lips!" ("Draft One" 00:47:15–00:47:45). In so many words, the doctor explains that his mad gestures are actually a common side effect of antipsychotic medication; and yet, passersby are unable to grasp this context, or so he implies. Following Edwin C. Hill, one might employ "a Fanonist term for this disorderly sounding: *ratés*—sonically charged backfires and failures" (14). Hill continues:

> *Ratés are* sonic breakdowns at the border between sound and text, the mythologies of Creole and black colonial speech as off script, the shocking sound of the colonial machine at work in black vernacular culture. The raté is a failure in time, a sonic symbol of slippage, excess, waste in the colonial machine and what Sartre calls its mental apparatus." (15)

Such sonic slippages present a form of "poetic cognition" in contrast to colonialist discourse and its knowledge schemas (15). Quoting the poet Audre Lorde, Bruce notes that anger is "full of information and energy," which is undoubtedly true of Dr. Chauvet's speech, if only his audience would listen closely (9). To hear him properly, one must be "versed in the idiom of madness—in the so-called rants, raves, rambles, slurs, outbursts, unseemly silences, and gibberish sounds typically coded as crazy" (47). On the contrary, the doctor knows that his audience is thoroughly unversed in, if not utterly averse to, his grammar. In one of the play's more direct statements on listening, Dr. Chauvet yet again exposes truths through mad logic: "Watch the walkers," he warns us, "the plugged-in ones, white earphones, they're downloading code" ("Draft One" 00:45:50–00:46:05). Though this admonishment could be understood as a trope of so-called paranoid schizophrenia, it is, in fact, much more than that: namely, a trenchant critique of the ideological and material systems from which we download the code that structures our listening.

The white earphones might therefore be understood as a resonant symbol for what sound studies scholar Jennifer Lynn Stoever calls the "sonic colour line," a concept built upon the visual equivalent introduced by the sociologist W.E.B. Du Bois. According to Stoever, the sonic colour line "produces, codes, and polices racial difference through the ear, enabling us to hear race as well as see it. It is a socially constructed boundary that racially codes sonic phenomena such as vocal timbre, accents, and musical tones" (11). In considering this boundary, what does it mean to listen through white earphones, if not to listen through white ears, or, in a more pointed sense, to listen through a piece of technology that serves as an ideological apparatus for white supremacy? In its resemblance to an earplug, the in-ear headphone, as such, perpetuates "selective listening habits," enabling white listeners to "tune out and/or mishear sounds of black agency" (205). As a result, Dr. Chauvet must shout even louder in order to penetrate the private acoustic space cultivated by the white listener who refuses to unplug.

As if to speak directly to this ideological barrier, the doctor describes a perceptual gap between his self-perception, and the way that others imagine him: "Baby, I ain't sick. I'm just smiling, just smiling, beguiling. I'm not defiling you. It's a fine line. I define the line, I define the line, the line, the line, the line, and how many steps it takes to cross the line, in between the line. You step on the line, or in the gap" ("Draft One" 00:47:40–00:47:55). Not only does Dr. Chauvet call attention to the existence of such a line, but, in doing so, he also employs a kind of mad syntax that has the potential to disrupt the listener's expectations. These conditioned responses are built around a set of co-constituting categories, including the fact that Dr. Chauvet is mad, Black, and unhoused. In other words, these categories become conflated within the white supremacist cultural imagination, or as Bruce puts it: "when black people get mad (as in *angry*), antiblack logics tend to presume they've gone mad (as in *crazy*)" (8).

Dr. Chauvet's frequent transitioning between lab coat and cardigan also accentuates the sonic colour line by revealing his double-voicedness. According to Stoever, "particular sounds are identified, exaggerated, and 'matched' to racialized bodies," thereby constructing aural stereotypes, along with the notion of "sounding black" (11). Dr. Chauvet steps on this line repeatedly as he code-switches between the "normative white speech patterns" of his clinical notes and the "black vernacular structures" of his mad monologues (246). It is important to remember, however, that the sonic colour line is a construct built around the matching of voices to bodies. By stepping back and forth across the line, Dr. Chauvet demonstrates its arbitrariness, and thus denaturalizes the practice of matching sound to skin.

In the process, he also dismantles "automatic associations of 'white' speech with truth-telling, reliability, and reason and 'black' speech with ignorance, entertainment, and fantasy" (167). By virtue of the fact that he embodies both doctor and patient, Dr. Chauvet resists racial and psychiatric essentialisms. Moreover, by presenting characters in multiple roles, Lena further confounds the logic of essences. For instance, in one scene midway through the play, the actor playing Ether dons a lab coat to treat Dr. Chauvet, inverting their respective roles. Yet, in an ironic turn, she attempts to reassert these roles, even though the audience is well aware of their doubling: "I'll take over," she says, "He's one of ours" ("Draft One" 00:50:15–00:50:20). She reminds him that he is a psychiatrist as if to suggest that someone in such a profession could not be mad, and this assumption is carried to its anticipated conclusion when Dr. Chauvet loses his job, at which point the writing quite literally appears on the wall via a projection: "You are no longer a psychiatrist, Franz" ("Draft One" 01:00:50–01:00:55).

On the contrary, in the midst of his madness, Dr. Chauvet proves himself to be a competent if not revolutionary psychiatrist. Under examination, he offers a tape cassette to the attending doctor, which contains his professional self-evaluation: "I have dictated clinical notes on my psyche, in relation to its particular history. I have described my cardinal symptoms: I hear voices—highly aggressive, hostile radio voices, with an inquisitorial character, carrying out a type of violent invasion" ("Draft One" 00:51:20–00:51:50). In this scene, Dr. Chauvet's voices are both sonified and personified: one takes the form of Frantz Fanon, who stands beside him as a ghostly presence, and the other is a booming voice that emanates from speakers in the room. As such, this scene's sound design is built around an audiovisual simulation of the doctor's madness, conveying a sense of what it might be like to see and hear, or look and listen, from his subject position. The low-pitched radio voice mocks and pathologizes him, calling him delusional, dysfunctional, prone to hallucinations, and an object of pity. At the same time, Fanon provides the subtext for the doctor's dialogue by giving voice to the unspoken, imploring the psychiatrist—and, by extension, the audience—to attend to missing contexts: "Listen to the gaps, the lapses. This is where you'll find me," he says ("Draft One" 00:52:15–00:52:20). Though one may raise questions about the representational politics of this scene's simulation of madness, Fanon's appeal to the listener suggests that there is more to understand beyond what is heard. To hear Dr. Chauvet's voices, in other words, is not to comprehend them automatically. Consequently, this scene also functions as a critique of simulations, since these counterfeit experiences can only ever reproduce the visible and the audible, and thus they tend to reinforce the hegemony of positivism.

The dramatic irony of this scene arises from the audience's access to the doctor's point of view and point of audition, whereas his psychiatrist—an empiricist—is stuck on the outside, looking and listening in. Unaware of the gaps in outward expression, the psychiatrist takes more interest in what the voices say than what they fail to express, addressing symptoms rather than root causes. When Dr. Chauvet describes a "violent invasion" of his psyche, for example, the psychiatrist does not seem to acknowledge the connotations of colonialism in his choice of words; however, Fanon fills in the gaps, so to speak, when he tells us that the doctor's voices belong to "the wretched, the damned, the dispossessed, the marginalized, the institutionalized, the racialized, the anaesthetized, the colonized" ("Draft One" 00:51:10–00:51:20). One of the violent invaders of Dr. Chauvet's psyche, the booming voice heard over loudspeakers, stands in for the pathologizing voice of psychiatry, which contests and delegitimizes the doctor's experience of voice hearing. Though Dr. Chauvet uses the term "voices," this invasive entity cuts him off immediately, saying: "Hallucinations, check" ("Draft One" 00:51:05–00:51:10). In the words of Maria Liegghio, a social worker and mental health researcher, mad persons are persistently denied the right to self-determination: "Alternative experiences of reality—defined as 'psychosis' or 'hallucinations'—become the rationale for the denial of their legitimacy as a knower. Rendered incompetent, persons are disqualified as legitimate knowers and lose their epistemic agency" ("Denial of Being" 118).

This is also true of the cassette that Dr. Chauvet tries to share with his psychiatrist. It is telling that he dictates his notes verbally onto tape, whereas the other doctors write on clipboards. His authority is delegitimized in two senses, then, in terms of the form of his madness, and the madness of his form. Crucially, the cassette never exchanges hands, which suggests a literal refusal to listen on the part of his psychiatrist. Dr. Chauvet puts the tape back in his jacket pocket after a few minutes, and it never reappears.

The play offers other contrasting moments, however, in which Dr. Chauvet's tapes are re-centred, and his self-knowledge is validated. To quote Liegghio once more: "If epistemic violence is to deny being, then the response to the violence is to construct ways that bring psychiatrized people back into existence" (119). One such response includes recognizing mad forms of expression and narration as valuable forms of self-expression, and not dismissing mad epistemologies as disordered, delusional, or dangerous. A good example of such acts of validation comes towards the end of the play, when Eduard reappears to join his father in a mad monologue. In recent years, a number of mad studies scholars have proposed methods of feeling *with* (La Marr Jurelle Bruce), listening *with* (Anna Harpin), and thinking *with* madness (Johanna Braun), and the aforementioned scene models all three of these orientations. In particular, Eduard embodies Bruce's notion of radical compassion towards madpersons when he dons a pair of headphones and mouths along to one of his father's tapes with the same fervour and conviction as the recording. To paraphrase Bruce: radical compassion, as a mad methodology, is not about collapsing interpersonal differences or becoming a tourist in someone else's lifeworld; rather, it is about moving alongside others in solidarity (10). It is precisely in this capacity that Eduard stands beside his father, Dr. Chauvet, who announces his own solidarity with historical figures in the Black radical tradition: "I stand among the tallest trees. I whisper through the wind, with my brothers Malcolm, Marcus, Martin, Miles and miles of yews, and hues of deep green" ("Draft One" 01:04:30–01:04:40). This is not only a statement of solidarity, of course, but also an appeal to the audience to recognize his mad testimony with the same sense of urgency, validity, and consequence as that proffered by such iconic figures. Slowly, Eduard begins to join in with his father's voice, echoing both his words and his gestures, culminating in them shouting in unison: "Black pain, red rain!" ("Draft One" 01:06:07–01:06:07). With this resonant gesture of solidarity, Eduard exemplifies both Black radical praxis, in Bruce's sense, and mad-positive listening. By replaying his father's tapes, and adopting the grammar of madness himself, Eduard resists the epistemic violence of the psychiatrist, who fails to recognize the narrative content of these cassettes as a valid form of self-knowledge. As per Liegghio, in the preceding scene, Dr. Chauvet is "reinstated as a legitimate knower with legitimate knowledge" by his son, who listens, feels, thinks, and resonates *with* madness in the very literal sense of re-sounding it verbally and physically. At the same time, it should be understood that Eduard echoes his father's madness without presuming any phenomenal overlap with Dr. Chauvet's lived experience. In other words, his performance is not an imitation or a simulation, but rather an act of solidarity.

Further emphasizing the significance of solidarity among listeners, Dr. Chauvet's vision of Fanon incarnate soon appears at a table, speaking into a microphone, where he delivers excerpts from his canonical 1959 essay "This Is the Voice of Algeria." In the essay, he describes the situation in French-colonial Algeria, in which colonizers took control of national radio broadcasts, such that Algerians were forced to listen to hostile French voices proclaiming military victory. In time, however, a new voice—"The Voice of Fighting Algeria"—emerged on the radio, around which entire towns would gather to listen, even as the French tried to jam Algerian radio signals. Paraphrasing Fanon, Lena writes:

> Each radio operator was engaged in a tactical battle with the enemy. Still, sometimes the French won, so the radio operator would fill in the gaps, reimagining events full of hope, heroic victories—whether they happened or not. The Algerians heard the voice. They all believed the voice. The voice carried them to victory. Their collective hallucination made history. And my patients? Well, their radio voices became friendly, encouraging, and protective against anxiety. The quality of the voice had changed. They all heard the voice: their voice. ("Draft One" 01:18:00–01:20:00)

With this speech, Lena reorients the play's focus away from individual pathology and towards collective struggle. In the context of Fanon's writing, Dr. Chauvet's so-called hallucinations, which he attributes to a tape recorder inside his head, carry a deeper historical and political resonance. Through this allusion to Algerian liberation, Lena once again draws attention to the colonial basis of medicalized madness. If there is a radio of sorts in Dr. Chauvet's mind, then we are led to ask who is responsible for its systematic jamming. The show's soundscape represents this jamming through occasional swells of electromagnetic interference, a repetitive hissing, beeping, or tapping noise. As a countermeasure, Ether goes about "lining the walls with foil" because it "blocks the signal completely" ("Draft One" 01:15:35–01:15:45). No doubt, this dynamic of jamming and anti-jamming is analogous to the sonic warfare undertaken by French and Algerian radio operators during the war, in Fanon's description. Implicit in this parallel is the sense that Ether and Dr. Chauvet's shared condition is indeed a form of colonial invasion and that their so-called delusions are in fact a reasonable response to systematic oppression. That Ether locates these invasive sounds within the actual walls of the institution, represented by partitions in the performance space, calls attention to the underlying foundations of structural violence perpetrated by colonial institutions. This is not to reduce madness to a metaphor, however, which would risk "evacuating madness of its lived complexity," to quote Bruce (15). As noted above, Fanon's essay demonstrates that the voice of the oppressor has material consequences, insofar as it changed the character of the Algerian listener's so-called hallucinations, which took on a negative valence under French colonialism, and acquired an increasingly positive valence as the insurgent voices of the revolution were amplified. Though the psychiatric label of "hallucination" may perpetuate stigma, Lena recuperates the term in the context of a collective will to struggle for mad liberation.

On one side, *Here are the Fragments* depathologizes voice hearing by exposing its roots in systemic injustice, which rightly pushes back against the medical model of madness. On the other side, however, the play's promotional material pursues the same outcome by universalizing madness—a strategy which tends to diminish lived experience by refusing to differentiate it from everyday life. One official writeup, for example, says the following: "People living with schizophrenia 'hear voices' and fear loss of control over their own thoughts and bodies. But how does any one of us actually separate internal and external voices?" ("Residency Page" par. 2). Though normalizing madness can work hand in hand with depathologizing so-called mental illness, the move towards universalization is stickier. According to disability and queer studies scholar Robert McRuer, the notion that "we are all disabled in some way" is a "complacent assertion" that allows an able-bodied, heterosexual, and psychonormative society to disregard "claims to rights and recognition" (157). Within the performance space of *Fragments*, such humanistic assumptions could indeed enable some of the more pernicious tendencies among listeners in the audience. The fantasy of an "idyllic oneness," as Bruce puts it, is a driving force behind disability simulations, which often entail a "smug projection of oneself into the position of another, thereby displacing that other" (10). To partake in this fantasy is to forget one's own listening position, and to feign ignorance about the ways that medicalized madness is discredited, degraded, incarcerated, pathologized, psychiatrized, policed, institutionalized, and otherwise oppressed. Unlike the smug listener's complacent projections, Dr. Chauvet's voice hearing is figured as a lived reality with material consequences. As McRuer notes: "The fact that some of us get beaten and left for dead tied to deer fences or that others of us die virtually unnoticed in underfunded and unsanitary group homes should be enough to highlight that the heterosexual/queer and able-bodied/disabled binaries produce real and material distinctions" (157). Such disheartening distinctions and appalling material consequences are borne out in the play's final scene, when Dr. Chauvet reappears, having had one of his arms amputated without his knowledge or consent: "I do not recall this amputation: the cause of it, the act of it. I do not recall it, Eduard. It is a fact I do not recall" ("Draft One" 01:24:00–01:24:15).

In discussing this scene, I would like to return to an earlier speech in which Dr. Chauvet asserts his intention to "devise a method of electrical extraction" in order to "transcend medicine" ("Draft One" 00:25:05–00:25:45). Here, we find Eduard and his father reunited in an attempt to do just that: to transcend institutional medical care by taking Dr. Chauvet's treatment into their own hands. Eduard has been researching an experimental psychiatric treatment called AVATAR therapy—a real treatment modality, invented by the psychiatrist Julian Leff in 2008—in which a "voice-hearer's experiences are brought into therapy in a new way, allowing a face-to-face interaction with a digital representation (avatar) whose speech closely matches the pitch and tone of the persecutory voice" (Craig et al. 32). Through this mediated interaction, voice-hearers are meant to gain "increased power and control within the relationship" by speaking back to a personified voice (32). Though their adoption of an official therapeutic model suggests further entrenchment in the hegemony of medicalized madness, it is important to acknowledge that Eduard and Dr. Chauvet take full ownership of the approach, engaging in something akin to "tactical biopolitics," as defined by interdisciplinary scholars Beatriz da Costa and Kavita Philip. In their radical appropriation of the AVATAR technology—not unlike the Algerian broadcasters in Fanon's account, who take back the radio—father and son engage in a mad praxis of self-knowledge, self-diagnosis, and self-treatment, in contrast to what Dr. Chauvet later calls "self-theft, self-repossession, self-storage" ("Draft One" 01:30:05–01:30:15). Despite this sense of self-determination, however, Dr. Chauvet remains sceptical about the institutional origins of this treatment, and rightfully doubts its safety. When asked about this, Eduard says: "It's up to you. I just did some research online," to which his father replies, "What line. Whose line?" ("Draft One" 01:25:00–01:25:10).

In the exchange that follows, Eduard goes about adjusting the avatar's appearance, projected onto a nearby wall: a white man named Dr. Robert, who is verbally abusive and has a severe, almost vampiric appearance. Once Eduard finds a close approximation of the man's image, he then speaks into a pitch-adjusted microphone in order to capture the man's persecutory voice. This proves too much for Dr. Chauvet, who tells his son, acting as the avatar, to stop shouting his name. According to a landmark research paper promoting AVATAR therapy, this interaction constitutes a trilogue "between therapist, patient, and a simulation of the auditory hallucination experienced by the patient" (32). Unlike other audiovisual simulations of madness, however, this one is different. Most notably, Dr. Chauvet controls the avatar's expressions by sculpting its appearance and scripting the content of its speech. The resulting simulation, then, abides by a standard of mad self-representation, albeit fictionalized.

Because of the play's psychiatric framing as a whole, the scene in question raises several issues. There is something uncomfortable, for example, about observing and overhearing someone in the privacy of therapy and to see such a treatment presented as though it were being demonstrated at a professional society. Though Lena does not present the audience with an image of false recovery, and indeed the play concludes on an open-ended note, Dr. Chauvet is nonetheless presented as a model patient. Across several large studies in AVATAR therapy, it is evident that things do not always go this smoothly: a large number of participants withdraw, some remain entirely unconvinced by the digital persona, and others experience indistinct voices that are not easily recreated. While a critical evaluation of this therapeutic model falls well outside the scope of the present chapter, it is not as though the play proceeds uncritically in this domain. In speaking back to his avatar, for instance, Dr. Chauvet shouts: "Your diagnostic dance is a fucking phobic ritual. Your ritual. I am turning remorse into accusation. I accuse you of diagnosing me" ("Draft One" 01:29:50–01:30:05). To the extent that it is hailed as a new frontier in psychiatry, virtual reality therapy is surely just one more step in this diagnostic dance.

As I have suggested, Dr. Chauvet radically appropriates this ritual, but it remains a psychotherapeutic ritual nonetheless. By accentuating the grey area here, Lena challenges the audience to reflect on strategies by which we represent mad subjectivity and the mechanisms behind such representations. No doubt, one of this scene's representational strengths is its transparency: Eduard stands in the open, speaking into a microphone, making live adjustments to the sound of his voice, listening and responding on the fly. Though the therapeutic model may rely, in part, on Dr. Chauvet's ability to conflate Eduard's voice with that of his persecutor, the audience can make no mistake about its constructedness. This is a representation of lived experience and not the thing itself. As such, there is no opportunity for fantasies of "oneness" to germinate, only a sense of "withness" when listening alongside Dr. Chauvet in solidarity. Here, Fanon's thoughts on the medium of radio might be applied more broadly to the play: "It is true to say that there never was, with respect to the radio, a pattern of listening habits, of audience reaction. Insofar as mental processes are concerned, the technique had virtually to be invented" (15).

With respect to *Fragments*, we can recognize the development of similar techniques and patterns, particularly in the case of avatar therapy, wherein Eduard and Dr. Chauvet revolutionize the technology by operating it autonomously, outside the bounds of institutional oversight.

Conclusion

In some sense, *Fragments* is a performance at odds with its own mode of presentation, given its simultaneous investment in staging psychiatric treatment and institutional critique, and yet the play is clearly aware of this friction, and takes the opportunity to seize on inherent contradictions and ambiguities. In *Fragments*, Lena continually prompts us to attend to unsounded truths that have fallen into the gaps and the cracks, and the invisible lines along which the act of listening becomes racialized and pathologized. If these are the fragments, then the play asks us to fill in the silences, like the missing time between scenes, in which a man's arm can disappear without explanation, and yet, by this point, we have heard enough to draw conclusions.

Building upon the case studies I have presented thus far, the next chapter takes a different form entirely—itself composed of fragments. Based on my engagement with the problematics of mad simulation, the "Notes on Mad Listening" that follow present an idiosyncratic approach to representing mad phenomenology, grounded in my own auditory experiences.

Notes

1. Adam Alston troubles this feature of immersive theatre where he writes about the trend of "dark dining." He writes: "Darkness in these restaurants functions as an environmental condition intended to defamiliarize the sensorium for sighted publics, but it is also presented as a (problematic) gateway to sight unseen through an Other's eyes. The success of dining in the dark restaurants like Dans Le Noir? rests on the appeal of difference and packaged otherness set at a safe distance from one's own everyday experiences, but that nonetheless facilitates fun flirtation with blindness' chimera. In other words, these restaurants build on a tension between ethics and aesthetics, juggling social responsibility and the profitable desire

for sensorial exploration among neophile consumers" ("Melting into Air" 65).

2. Another key observation comes from Julie Beth Napolin, who notes that resonance and vibration can act as mediums for "atrocious content" (*Fact of Resonance* 193). One need only to compare and contrast two different public speeches and their aftereffects to recognize the most glaring issue with resonance as a political-affective strategy.
3. Furthermore, according to Hannah Zeavin in *The Distance Cure: A History of Teletherapy* (2021), Sigmund Freud insisted that "the relationship between the analyst and the patient is like that of two persons communicating by telephone," and that the talking cure was based on unpacking symptomatic speech (54).

CHAPTER 5

Notes on Mad Listening

In her famous treatise on camp, Susan Sontag introduces the topic by saying that many things have been named but not described. This chapter concerns the opposite: something described but not named. I am inclined to call it "mad listening." For me, this umbrella term encapsulates a wide range of neurodivergent orientations to sound, from hallucination to phobia to synesthesia to other experiential modes that you will not find in the DSM.

Mad listening should not be thought of as an essentialism or a universalism. This chapter is, most of all, a personal history: part positionality statement and part "autobiographical topography," to borrow a term from the film critic Kier-La Janisse.[1] One could also call it autoethnography or autotheory, though I am not necessarily trying to reinvent either of these wheels, only trying to balance my thoughts on them. Following the anthropologist Kathleen Stewart and her personal-as-political theorization of ordinary affects, I am presenting this chapter as a loose assemblage of notes, riffs, anecdotes, vignettes, and fragments, with the goal of forming a noncoherent "mass of resonances" (6). To that end, it would be most accurate to say that I am interested in conjuring an atmosphere rather than an argument—provocations and attunements and residues rather than "evaluative critique" (4). Much like Stewart, I want to create a critical framework that is not dependent on closure and clarity.

M. Tomkinson, *Sound and Sense in Contemporary Theatre*,
https://doi.org/10.1007/978-3-031-78034-9_5

Though my approach is intensely personal, I hope it is this very quality that makes this collection of extraordinary affects and resonances palpable. Film scholar Miklós Kiss argues that "an escalating subjectivity should not mellow our (scholarly) ideals concerning argumentative precision and accountability," and yet "one should not reject the rise of subjectivity off-hand, as it might be a key to evolving a more human Humanities" (n.pag). Though this chapter arrives last in the book, it does not purport to be conclusive, nor does it uphold "the personal" as a basis for collective knowledge. At the very least, some of the embodied or experiential knowledge shared in this chapter offers a counterdiscourse to standard academic research, which tends to problematize first-person writing as undisciplined and unrigorous.

Autotheory can assume many different shapes, but generally it takes the form of highly subjective and performative writing that combines self-expression with so-called expert philosophical analysis. This experimental form of critical engagement is a vital counterbalance within mad studies because of the ways that psychiatric professionals throughout history have ignored the personal contexts of their patients. Moreover, academia has a history of legitimizing certain kinds of knowledge at the expense of others—namely, reason over unreason, objectivity over subjectivity, and so on. Mad studies scholar Kathryn Church puts it this way: "the lived experience of madness [is] a fundamental form of human knowledge" that has been "suppressed and subordinated over time" (171). Autotheory, then, is one potential form of counter-discursive knowledge that can support mad artists and academics in resisting the dominance of psy-centred ways of thinking.

This chapter takes a mad first-person standpoint, drawn from my own experience of obsessive–compulsive disorder, depression, and generalized anxiety, among other crazed aspects of my unruly bodymind that evade diagnosis. Challenging the power that diagnoses hold—but not negating their importance for some people—I propose alternative ways of retheorizing these idiosyncratic experiences, through abstract intensities such as "stickiness." By depathologizing and de-medicalizing madness in favour of minor affects, my goal is to emphasize the persistent ambiguities and slippages of auditory perception that are not so easy to taxonomize. As such, I aim to chart a poetics of the perceptual glitch in relation to mad listening, without the footholds and straightjackets of psychiatric terminology. Linking mad praxis to other intersections of radical unreasoning, this essay presents further challenges to audist and phonocentric assumptions, which tend to abound where listening subjectivities are concerned.

This chapter attempts to illustrate my lifelong experience of non-normative listening, which sometimes takes the form of an active practice (in listening "against the grain" of neurotypicality) and, at other times, comes on suddenly in a moment of disturbance and disorientation. To quote feminist and queer studies scholar Sara Ahmed: "Disorientation could be described here as the 'becoming oblique' of the world, a becoming that is at once interior and exterior" (163). Ahmed insists that it is a matter of irresolvable tension as to whether "the strangeness is in the object or in the body that is near the object" (163). Following Lisa Blackman, a majority of the scenarios described below are concerned with "anomalous experiences or threshold phenomena," wherein distinctions are unsettled between inner and outer, near and far, real and imaginary, material and immaterial (para. 6). If such thresholds are spaces of epistemic uncertainty, as Blackman suggests, then to listen madly might sometimes take the form of inhabiting such indeterminacy, perhaps even embracing it. Though threshold phenomena are part of everyday experience, this does not mean that everyone is equally attuned or sensitized to them, nor at all times.

I have been fortunate to find support for this project (both financial and otherwise) from the University of British Columbia's Public Scholars Initiative. The audio version of this chapter, which the PSI supported, is a valuable part of my larger research project because it legitimizes forms of knowledge production and distribution other than the standard academic essay, and such a non-traditional approach aligns with the methodological goals of mad studies and disability studies in resisting sanist and ableist ways of writing, thinking, and knowing.[2] This chapter also allows me to wear two hats at once as an artist-scholar. In effect, I see this arts-based research as a comprehensive "thinking-through-sound" of this book as a whole, both supplementing and being supplemented by my primary research concerns, foremost of which is the question of how mad auralities have been staged in performance.

My autotheoretical research not only connects with mad performance theory but also aims to connect to mad activism. In keeping with the "public" aspect of the aforementioned initiative, I hope this audio work will be relevant to a general audience—especially other mad-identified artists. The audio component is an example of arts-based research, rooted in my experiences as a mad-identified scholar and my early career as a professional sound designer. My hope is that the inclusion of a more populist form of life writing in this book will make the project more accessible as a whole. The use of arts-based methods has been fundamental, in this regard, to disability and mad studies broadly. Mad activist-scholars from Toronto Metropolitan University, including Jenna Reid, Sarah N. Snyder, Jijian Voronka, Danielle Landry, and Kathryn Church, have proposed "mad art as a way to think through aesthetic values; as a tool to theorize issues central to the emergent field of mad studies; and as a practice that blurs the line between the academy and the larger (mad) community" (269). These authors suggest that mad art is, in many ways, fundamentally at odds with the neoliberal university, if not in a "turbulent relation" (261).

Though I have been fortunate to find a receptive audience within the university for this kind of work—and also well aware of how my privilege means that my perspective is seen as valid—it is important to recognize the limitations that are still in place. Whatever is defiant about madness is inevitably consumed under the "inclusionism" of the university, as Reid et al. have underlined. By one measure, arts-based research subverts traditional research and writing conventions; but, by another measure, it is subsumed as an additional skill to bolster academic job applications or treated as supplemental material to the "real" work of close analysis. In its cooptation, mad arts within the academy stands to lose some of its potential to "provoke, defy, and resist" (263). For the sake of preserving these efforts, it is essential that the "activist aesthetic objects come first [...] before they are later written-up into academic articles" (267). If this resonates with you, then feel free to skip the rest of this academic preamble and go directly to the notes below, or the audio, linked in the chapter's endnotes.

If you are still here, then I wanted to say something about the notable dangers of disclosure within academia. Because this project draws heavily on personal narrative, I accept certain risks of disclosure, though these risks are proportional to my privilege. So far, I have been privileged to be able to do this kind of work with enthusiasm and encouragement from my peers, let alone a lack of serious repercussions due to stigma. It has not always been easy, however, and I have tried many times to break the academic mould over the years, only to have my mind, body, and spirit broken instead. There are innumerable challenges that come with negotiating madness within the academy, where there are few opportunities to share these experiences in an unguarded way. Though I cannot speak for anyone else, I hope to signal-boost other critical voices, to welcome other mad-affirmed narratives, to open up space for further discussions and disruptions within academic practice, to question the processes and forms by which we produce knowledge, and to challenge the criteria by which particular kinds of knowledge are deemed valid.

Writing about brain fog as a cripistemology, gender, and queer studies scholar Mel Y. Chen says that "cognitive variation [...] represents the near unthinkable for academia," and personal experience testifies to this (177). In contrast to scholarly comprehensiveness, Chen speaks of partial knowledge as a means of resisting sanism. A renewed commitment to partiality exposes the fantasy of the solitary thinker and reaffirms the value of shared cognitive labour (179). Quoting a conference presentation by disability and queer studies scholar Robert McRuer, Chen defines cripistemologies as "seriously twisted ways of knowing in the current global order" (McRuer qtd. in Chen 173). The aim of this audio essay is to develop a twisted cripistemology of sorts, a highly partial and provisional perspective on madness and sensory knowledge working in opposition to sanism and stigma. Thank you for reading and/or listening.

Notes on Mad Listening

1. Wherever you are right now, I invite you to pause and listen, taking a moment to situate yourself. Whenever you are ready, try to pick out five sounds or felt-vibrations in your environment. A dripping faucet. The humming of an appliance. A garbage truck backing up. Trees shaking in the wind. The call of an unfamiliar bird. Dull footsteps from the upstairs apartment. A buzzing off in the distance that could be a blender, or a circular saw, or a vacuum, or a pressure washer. It is hard to say. Doubt always creeps in. [Overdub from Peter Brook's 1967 film adaptation of *Marat/Sade*: "Why is everything so confused now. Everything I wrote or spoke was considered and true. Each argument was sound. And now, doubt. Why does everything sound false?" (1:31:15–1:31:4589)].
2. Perhaps the most famous of all mad listeners is the "very dreadfully nervous" protagonist of Edgar Allen Poe's short story, "The Tell-Tale Heart" (121). After murdering a man, he is driven to confess his crime because of an unsettling sound that torments him from beneath the floorboards, where the body lies. He describes

the sound as a low pulse, like that of a watch wrapped in cotton. In this story, Poe describes an insect called the deathwatch beetle, a critter known for making a very distinct hissing noise which resembles a heartbeat. The composer and sound theorist François J. Bonnet describes this fictional listening situation as an example of "panic listening." According to Bonnet, hallucinations arise from the moment when "affects, desires, and phobias act directly upon perception, subjecting it to their own prerogatives" (170). If those five sounds you noticed earlier are still perceptible, what do they sound like now? What kind of affects, desires, and phobias are present? In what ways do they shape the noisy world around you, and vice versa?

3. In the early summer of this year, one of my neighbours backed over and flattened a crow with his truck—gruesome and heartbreaking, I know. For weeks afterwards, two more crows made relentless alarm calls in the tree outside our window—a much harsher cawing than usual, paired with strange dances upon the branches. I learned that this was an elaborate funerary ritual of sorts. Still, the sound was unbearable to me, and I entertained a number of desperate measures. Maybe we could face some speakers out the window and shout them away, like an auditory scarecrow (notwithstanding the environmental ethics of upsetting nature's acoustic balance in this way, but I hope you will forgive me). It was only a few hours later that I had completely forgotten about these schemes. At noon, I logged onto my online therapy appointment. I was having—still am having—a tough time with dissociation. My therapist and I talked about grounding techniques, strategies for reconnecting to the physical world, being present in sensation. Just then, as if conjured by thought, a bald eagle let out a majestic peal above our apartment. I could hear the crows battling with it, probably as it tried to raid their nest. The high-pitched piping of the eagle was impossible to ignore. Both of us took off our headphones and listened intently. The sound went on for a few minutes like that, and I remember thinking: O.K. universe, what message are you trying to send me? There was something deeply earnest and spiritual about the moment, accompanied by embarrassing tears of wonder. My embarrassment was about to multiply, however—and you might have already guessed where this is going. Some germ of wisdom concerning my dissociation was extracted

from the eagle scenario: *when in doubt, return to the birds, return to the birds, return to the birds*. I logged off with this thought circling profoundly in my head, stumbling into the living room like someone struck by a miracle. "Wasn't that incredible?" I said to my partner. I asked if she had seen it. She had no idea what I was talking about. "The eagle!" I said. Outrageous laughter ensued. Behind her, facing out the window: a portable speaker, connected to a laptop with the YouTube video still pulled up: "10 Hours of Eagle Sounds." For such a sophisticated organ as the ear, it is remarkably susceptible to mishearings. I could have sworn that the eagle was not a speaker in the opposite corner of my house but a creature of blood-and-bone whose piercing voice was conducted cleanly through the air and not bent through electrical circuits and distorted by apartment walls. Mad listening makes fools of us all.

4. To listen madly, for me, is to listen to things on the edge of perception—the faint buzz of a dimmer switch or the sound of distant traffic through closed windows. Sound studies scholar Brian Kane reads one of Franz Kafka's short stories, "The Burrow," as an example of acousmatic listening, which refers to sounds whose sources cannot be determined (147). In Kafka's story, a mole tries to locate the source of a humming noise that reverberates throughout its underground channels. This mole comes up with seven possible explanations for the sound, but none of them are substantiated. Mad listening exists here, in the uncertain and uncomfortable threshold of unknowingness.
5. The period of stillness before bed is often one of heightened awareness, when my entire being is full of leftover energies from the day. Residual neurons seem to fire like the tiny pings of a warm engine after it is turned off. As a light and restless sleeper, I have become dependent on a steady drone of brown noise to help me shut off. Sometimes, when I am lying awake, I hear hushed voices, and sometimes faint music, emanating from within the static. But I am always less than sure that these sounds are coming from the speaker and not, in fact, someone in the next room or a conversation on the street far below. Certainty is not part of the equation. On few occasions, I have heard looping melodies that I am unable to distinguish as mind sounds or room sounds. The noise machine seems to create a bridge between these two spaces of mind and room. When this happens, I usually become quite anxious. It does

not help that my partner never hears what I hear. I turn off the noise machine to see if these sounds might be coming from another apartment, or I put my head right next to the speaker in an attempt to locate these phantasms. Voices speak or sing in the soft hum. There are words, but not intelligible words. My first guess is that some kind of stray signal is cutting through, not unlike the way that old dental fillings would sometimes pick up radio signals. But there is also a long history of people hearing ghosts in the machine, otherwise known as Electronic Voice Phenomena (EVP). The parapsychologist Konstantin Raudive, a student of Carl Jung, collected thousands of recordings of white noise, from which he extracted an abundance of uncanny phrases. According to Raudive, "The voices often maintain that we do nothing but sleep. This is repeated under many different circumstances" (*Breakthrough* 270). One of these radio voices, speaking in a combination of Swiss German and Latvian, was reported to have said to the experimenters: "Good day, we are the mad ones here" (111).

6. According to an experimental theory collective called The Occulture, "whether phenomena such as EVP are real or not is never really the question, entrenched as they are in the manifestation of differing hallucinatory registers of possibility" (111). The authors suggest that even the biggest EVP sceptic "may also be playing with pareidolia"—a term that refers to a form of heightened pattern recognition wherein people tend to find meaning in random stimuli (111). The EVP sceptic finds a negative meaning, or what The Occulture calls a "negative hallucination" (111). In other words, the sceptic hears nothing but white noise because this is the only pattern that such a person can recognize. By turning hallucination inside out in this way, perhaps we might remove some of the stigma and pathologization from voice hearing.
7. If you were online in 2018, you probably heard about the "Yanny or Laurel" phenomenon. A short recording features a man pronouncing the word "Laurel," which can also be heard as "Yanny." Remarkably, the general population seems to be divided fifty-fifty on which one of these words is most audible. This glitch in the Matrix exposed not just the perceptual instability within us, but also the perceptual gaps between us, reminding us that listening is highly contextual and provisional, dependent on countless factors such as age, speaker placement, musical background,

cultural context, and so on. We have a tendency to think that what we hear is a mirror of something concrete in the world, but this is not so. As one study from *Current Biology* puts it: "Sensory information is always fragmentary and noisy, so by nature it cannot unambiguously reflect the state of the world at every instant. Rather, perception must make inferences, which are often unconscious. These inferences draw prior information from past experience, be it long-term expertise or immediate context" (Pressnitzer et al. 741). Another study from Stanford suggests that 2% of the top 10,000 words in the English language could be polyperceivable, including pairs such as frank/strength, claimed/framed, settle/civil, or floral/family (Chandra et al. 1). If polyperceivability is so prevalent in spoken language, then perhaps to listen madly is to recognize that all hearing involves mishearing and that the binary of mad and sane is confounded by the persistent presence of one inside the other.

8. People like to say that certain noises "drive them mad." I for one have no problem with nails on a chalkboard, whereas the very mention of this auditory image might make you wince. Recently, I read an article in the Harvard Health Blog that describes rain as a neutral sound, as compared to the disturbance of a crying baby ("Misophonia"). But really, if you think about it, there is no neutral sound, no neutral rain. You can bet that somewhere on the news, a meteorologist is shouting over a thunderstorm. In my experience, neutral-seeming sounds can be the most unpleasant. Take this scenario, for example: I recall sitting with my friend at the breakfast table one morning as he ate a plain bagel with jam. It was not that he chewed with his mouth open, but that the muffled chomping of his cheeks was unbearable for reasons that are impossible to explain. The sound of the bagel overtakes one's entire body. I imagine it like a lifebuoy thrown over my head, pinning my arms to my sides. I feel trapped inside this sound. It is annoying enough to have been invented by someone who knows what they are doing. The hair on the back of my neck stands up, and I want to flee the room. I try to concentrate on other things, but the sound overrides my efforts. It bypasses my ears and goes straight into my spine. If I try to ignore it, I am drawn deeper into it. The background refuses to stay backgrounded. In moments such as this one, it almost feels like the most trivial stimuli could leap out and

kill you. The house is full of potential triggers. A dripping faucet, a ticking clock. Just typing this makes my heart speed up, and I feel the urge to retreat to the soundproof room I have constructed in my mind, the room that no sound can enter, not even the neutral rain.

9. Even if a sound were neutral, it can quickly lose its supposed neutrality through repetition, which is a formal archetype—if not a cliché—of mad sound. The TV Tropes website, for example, has pages devoted to the "Madness Mantra" ("All work and no play makes Jack a dull boy") and Incessant Music Madness ("This is the song that never ends. Yes it goes on and on, my friends"). Whether we are talking about looping or chanting or muttering or stuttering, the idea of madness is often implicit. In Tom Murphy's 1985 play *Bailegangaire* (pronounced "balya-gon-goyra"), an elderly woman repeats the same story to her granddaughter every night without finishing it. The incessant repetition of the unfinished story starts to wear on her until, at last, she says that she is going crazy. She pauses to reflect on this statement, however, and decides that she is not crazy after all. Or rather, it is implied that she is not the crazy one. Her grandmother Mommo speaks in crazy-sounding sentences: "The aspect silver of moon an' stars reflecting off the new impossibility" (79). One reviewer of this play, Bruce Weber, describes the grandmother as a "maddening and enraging" storyteller, whose incoherence is "tough to tolerate" (n.pag). "There's a pretentiousness," says Weber, "about the playwright's insistence in letting Mommo try the audience's patience as well as her granddaughters'" (n.pag). Let's agree that Weber's reaction is uncharitable at best. I use this example of *Bailegangaire* to model one of the ethical demands of mad listening—namely, that incoherence is not simply to be tolerated, but also celebrated. To listen madly is to listen patiently with madness, and not against it.

10. The prospect of listening with another person by means of sharing their sensory subjectivity is nonetheless a fantasy. Allow me to offer an example from my personal life: I am among a small subset of people with so-called obsessive–compulsive disorder who experiences something called sensorimotor obsessions or "Somatic OCD." This term refers to the tendency to fixate on autonomic bodily processes such as blinking and breathing to the point where

they become distressing. Another common point of fixation is the heartbeat, feeling stuck in a constant awareness of one's pulse—the way it sounds and the way it feels, in combination. Like Poe's tell-tale heart, this noise rises above all other noises, forcing its way into every interaction and every conversation, to the point where one wants to rip up floorboards. I could include a sound effect here to demonstrate to you what this experience feels like—a subtle pulse in your left ear—but what would this communicate? Would this validate my experience, or cheapen it? After all, the heartbeat I am describing is not just a sound but an interpretation of a sound. As François J. Bonnet puts it, "the sound-object must be understood at once as the object formed by listening [...] and as the *objectal projection* of listening's desire" (136). For this reason, aural experiences of madness cannot be easily represented, since auditory simulations of such phenomena tend to lack what Bonnet calls "the affective import and the signifying framework" (140). For me, OCD is one such framework (albeit a top-down diagnostic one whose voluntary adoption carries a set of risks). It is not such a deterministic fact that it overrides the social construction of madness, but it nonetheless plays an active role in shaping the objects of my aural attention. To share one's listening, then, must involve an understanding of the frameworks inside of which certain sounds reverberate differently inside each of us, much like spiders and their webs.

11. I have always been sensitive to sound. Even the smallest noises can make me jump. I am told that the startle reflex comes from the inner ear, where the tensor tympani muscle experiences an acoustic reflex in the presence of particular sounds. To hear oneself hearing—to feel the musculature of one's ear responding to sound—is an incredibly strange and unnerving experience. In my former job as a cashier, I would have to count the register at the end of the day, flicking coins into a plastic tray. Every time I would flick a coin, my inner ear would click like a retractable pen, accompanied by a dull noise—always a microsecond delay, too, between the coin toss and the click, an echo-like call and response. There was a certain satisfaction to the reflex, but also an immense fatigue, like listening to a ball-peen hammer gently tap an anvil. I would play with this clicking effect until I had expended its novelty, much in the same way that one's tongue keeps returning

to a sore tooth. The composer Maryanne Amacher suggested that people themselves become instruments as the ear has the potential to both receive and emit sound ("Psychoacoustic Phenomena" 10). To have one's sense perception inverted in this way can be wonderfully destabilizing. I listen with my inner ear to my inner ear—a strange aural Möbius strip. I become a lightning rod, a feedback loop, a sound experiencing itself.

12. When I was twelve or thirteen, I went through an Oliver Sacks phase, absorbing his dubious but riveting clinical tales. I was particularly compelled by his description of a man named Stephen who dreamed he was a dog and woke up with a heightened sense of smell. This was one of my first indications that the horizons of perception should not be taken for granted and that they can stretch and transform at any moment. Within a few months of reading this account, I experienced such a transformation first-hand. One afternoon, my friends and I went trekking through a peat bog just off the highway. Somewhere on our way out of the woods, as we tiptoed across river stones or clambered over a concrete drainage pipe, my hearing underwent a tenfold increase in volume, which I experienced as a rapid lightning-strike event. The gentle quietude of nature suddenly became noisier than the busiest intersection, painfully and supernaturally loud, and there was nothing I could do to reverse it. The slow-moving creek, not more than a stagnant trickle, now sounded like whitewater rapids, a high-decibel assault. I lagged behind my friends, desperately tugging on my earlobes as though they were on–off switches. Regretfully, I pretended like nothing was wrong at that moment. I hid the suffering. My friend's voices, their whispers even, sounded like vivid distortions. I tolerated this as best I could, and no one seemed to be able to tell that something was going on within me. Obviously, my auditory system had changed somehow. Some kind of gate had been left open, some threshold crossed. We parted ways, and I cupped my ears the entire way home. Coming up my driveway, I remember uncupping my ears and opening the front door as slowly as if I were defusing a bomb. Upon closing it behind me, the latch met the doorframe like a firing pin hitting a bullet. I ran upstairs, jumped into bed, cried softly, and fell asleep. When I woke up, it was like nothing had happened, and I was relieved that the bedsheets sounded like bedsheets.

13. There is a constant ringing within me. I first noticed it while wearing a pair of noise-cancelling headphones. Within the muffled silence of the earpads, I noticed all sorts of subtle impingements, the most prominent of which was a small, piercing tone in the upper range of my hearing. This tone comes and goes in waves. Sometimes it sounds tinny and shrill and other times it sounds like a weak drone, like a phone left off the hook. I can hear the sound change as I think about its changing nature. Like any bothersome sensation, the more I try not to feel it, the more it grows. The ringing seems to intensify at night, but this is really just its reemergence from beneath the clamour of the day. Earplugs do not help. If anything, they trap you inside with this annoying pest—this guest who refuses to leave, this kettle that is always boiling, this mosquito that lives in my head and soundtracks my life. Though the sound lives primarily in my left ear, I can feel it resonate throughout my entire body like a nerve being pinched and iced. It was only when the ringing started to keep me awake at night that I decided to see an audiologist. He told me to wait three months and come back if it did not go away. That was almost a year ago, now. Last night I woke up with the same sensation, another hijacking. A body being yoked to an object to which it does not want to be bound. I have surprised myself with patience and tolerance and appreciation for this sound, its musicality, and its beauty. I throw my head back in mad laughter at the sound's vibrating mockery. I have compassion for my captor, since it cannot be anything other than it is. But any silver lining is liable to tarnish after hours of wear. I toss and turn in anguish and would trade anything to make this sound go away. I picture a crucifix with the ears dripping blood.
14. Earworms are strange little mind vampires. They are stickier than other songs, and if you hear one, it might play on a mental loop for hours, possibly even years. Like con artists, they have tricks to get in your head. They are often tiny splinters of melody, and like splinters, they have a tendency to lodge under your skin. They are the musical equivalent of the hiccups, an involuntary and ephemeral glitch. Some of these earworms come from songs you actually know but cannot place—I am thinking of an insistent tune that I hummed for a couple of months that turned out to be a version of "Ticket to Ride" by the Carpenters. Like other self-reflexively

earwormy songs, such as Kylie Minogue's "Can't Get You Out of My Head," this one speaks of repetitious sad thoughts. As such, it has been expertly crafted to exploit a breach in one's consciousness, since the lyrics are pre-encoded as a repetitive thinking pattern. And because the song slowly fades out on a repeated phrase, failing to arrive at a final resolution, the melodic hook sinks even deeper. Fortunately, this is one of my more tolerable earworms. If they are good songs, like this one, then it is like a nice little bird that lands on my shoulder and sings to me. But if they are bad songs, then the earworm is like a gremlin that jumps on my back and zaps my brain repetitively with an electric cattle prod. Either way, the earworm becomes louder than anything else. It becomes everything I am, filling my world completely. It loops and loops and loops and, in its looping, it epitomizes the notion of going loopy. Earworms are one heightened phenomenon of my particular affliction; my mind is a sticky trap, lined with Krazy Glue. But, eventually, even the stickiest of traps will dry up. Even the stickiest songs, even the stickiest thoughts, will release their hold.

15. Are earworms an empowerment or a vulnerability? Philosopher and sound studies scholar Eldritch Priest suggests that they can be both a technique of resistance and a product of contemporary capitalism's demands on one's nervous system. For Priest, earworms can be a form of inutile thinking—and thus an affront to cognitive capitalism—but they can also be a form of affective labour. In either case, he frames them not as a mental pathology but as a side effect of living in a "chaotic media sphere" that constantly places demands on one's attention ("Eldritch Priest" n.pag). As such, Priest wonders if the earworm could be thought of as a means of re-capturing one's attention "from the constant tug of outward distractions" (n.pag). The critical theorist Tang Yan similarly looks for liberatory potential in the earworm. According to Yan, "being worm-ized is being weak and abject and mad. Being worm-ized is being happy and strong and dancing like a dragon. Being worm-ized is being free from making a decision" (152). Priest goes even further to suggest that earworms "might actually arrest the flow of desire," by reclaiming a person's attention from capitalist forces of distraction ("Eldritch Priest" n.pag). Though this is a compelling idea, I am not convinced that negative attention is inherently better than positive distraction. There are some earworms so corrosive

that I cannot even bring myself to name them, in case they latch on to me again—and when this happens, I am thankful for distractions, and long for them. If earworms could in any way pose a threat to the capitalist system that deploys them in the first place, perhaps it is in the sense of having laid awake all night, singing songs by the Carpenters, too tired to perform at one's job the next day. This formula requires a person to be expendable, however, in order to submit completely to wormization. Is it worth surrendering the sovereignty of one's attention for this political gesture? Perhaps not.

16. Mad listening is a multisensory if not synaesthetic affair, wherein the rationalist segmentation of the senses does not obtain.[3] Sometimes, when I am wearing my headphones and I hear an unexpected high-frequency pitch, like the highest possible harmonic overtones played on a violin, I start to notice a burning smell in my nostrils, as though my brain has been poked with a hot needle and some of the smoke is coming out my nose. Researchers call this "smound," a portmanteau of smell and sound.
17. If the ear is the dominant sensory organ of hearing, then to listen madly is to detach hearing from this default site and locate it elsewhere—in other words: a non-cochlear listening. In the composer Peter Ablinger's 2010 piece, *Palastmusik für Infra- und Ultraschall* (2010), a wooden bench is fitted with special loudspeakers that produce sub-auditory sound, which listeners experience as vibrations in their bodies ("Window Piece"). More recently, the composer Christine Sun Kim produced a work called *Elevator Pitch* (2019), which was "inspired by Kim's childhood memories of crowding elevators with her Deaf friends, and shouting so loudly that they could feel the vibrations of each others' voices" ("Elevator Pitch"). Another example comes from sound studies scholar David Cecchetto, who describes wearing a pair of shoes with microphones attached, with audio signals being routed in real time to headphones, thereby creating a sense of listening through one's feet ("Listening, Computation, and the Afterlife of Data"). Cecchetto's account resonates with a passage from Daniel Paul Schreber's journals, published in 1903 as *Memoirs of My Nervous Illness*, in which he describes two little men whose voices he can hear in his feet (135). Though the former example should not serve as a direct simulation of the latter, both cases of foot-based hearing

support a mad agenda. Whether through a bench or elevator or shoes, to listen from a non-dominant point of reference is to unsettle one's given mode of listening, or what Ablinger calls "the spoon-fed patterns of human perception" ("Palastmusik").

18. One also thinks of eye music or *Augenmusik*, visual scores that cannot be played by any classical standard. I remember sitting in the car as a child and waiting for the ticking of our turn signal to synchronize with the blinker of the car ahead—or watching the second hand of my old Seiko watch, with its fluorescent hands, tracing time's inaudible rhythm. These are but the simplest forms of seeing sound. In 1995, the poet Ella Mae Lentz conceived an ASL poem called "Eye Music," about the visual rhythms created by passing telephone poles along the roadside, a sine wave of rising and falling wires ("Signed Music"). This form of visual listening is not inherently mad, but it shares a key feature of mad listening in its resistance to audist assumptions. If mad listening is to be a political strategy, then it must intersect with Deaf culture and other non-normative auralities in challenging stigma and expanding the definition of listening itself.
19. Mad listening has an affinity for unwieldy compositions, repurposed and reappropriated technologies, imaginary sounds, and speculative instruments. As for the unwieldy, consider the famous pianist Éric Satie's 1893 composition, "Vexations," which asks the performer to repeat a motif eight hundred and forty times. As for acts of détournement or creative repurposing, consider the media artist Nam June Paik's 1963 installation, *Random Access Music* (1963), which disassembles a cassette deck and allows the listener to wave the playback head over numerous lines of tape that have been glued to the wall in a weblike pattern. Also consider the composer Raven Chacon's 2015 performance called *Report*, "a composition scored for an ensemble playing various caliber firearms" which seeks to turn instruments of power and violence "into mechanisms for musical resistance" (n.pag). As for sounds that do not exist, see the minimalist composer Tom Johnson's collection of unplayable scores in his 1974 book *Imaginary Music*. And as for the speculative, see the experimental musician Tom Mudd's 2019 album *Brass Cultures* which was created with "digital models of physically impossible brass instruments" (n.pag). Each of these works radically disobeys the laws of listening, creating a

possible space for mad subjectivity—a liberated space of ambiguity, excess, and paradox.

20. Put it this way: mad sounds prompt mad listening. Things that are hard to say are often difficult to hear. Songs that are hard to sing are often difficult to harmonize with. Music that is hard to play is often difficult to follow.
21. In his book *How to Go Mad Without Losing Your Mind: Madness and Black Radical Creativity*, interdisciplinary scholar and critical theorist La Marr Jurelle Bruce listens to the singer and rapper Lauryn Hill in the context of her fast-paced live performances. "Hill's manic delivery," writes Bruce, "like her occasionally hoarse vocals and cacophonous arrangements, resists *easy listening*. She solicits a nimble, attentive, difficult listening instead" (212). Here, Bruce does not romanticize mania but treats Hill's music as an example of "madtime," a mad temporality that the author situates within Black expressive culture and conceptualizes as a form of resistance against anti-Black admonishments to pursue justice slowly and reasonably (206). In another chapter, Bruce writes about a mad jazz musician named Buddy Bolden, who is thought to have invented jazz, but whose life is scarcely documented. Bruce shares an anecdote from one of Bolden's greatest fans: fellow jazz musician Ferdinand "Jelly Roll" Morton, who claimed that Bolden was such a loud cornetist that his playing could be heard from twelve miles away, though this reminiscence defies the laws of physics and human physiology (42). The author upholds Morton's story as an example of Black radical creativity in the face of normative psychiatry, which seeks to denigrate, pathologize, and discredit such fantastical accounts. "Upon reading Morton's twelve-mile testimony," writes Bruce, "a devout rationalist might dismiss it as deliberate fabrication, or a failure of memory, or a miscalculation of distance, or perhaps the product of delusion" (42). The task of mad methodology, according to Bruce, is to take such accounts seriously and to find metaphysical truths in them, if not physical ones—to listen as an affirming earwitness to sounds that exceed reason and distance and probability. To paraphrase Bruce, the truth is that Bolden's cornet call "echoed across epochs" to influence future artists and writers such as himself (43).

22. Following Bruce, we might discern other instances "where disclosures of pathology are also articulations of philosophy" (60). Take, for example, the phenomenon of the talking breast pump. According to medieval studies scholar Christine Cooper-Rompato, "many women who pump their breast milk report that their pumps speak repeated words or phrases" (182). She describes these phrases as auditory illusions or examples of pareidolia (not unlike the electronic voice phenomena I mentioned earlier). Many of the phrases that Cooper-Rompato documents involve one bisyllabic word or expression repeated over and over again, such as "nipple," "get her," "fresh milk," "not yours," or "pump me" (186). "Several mothers," she tells us, "report hearing taunts about their insufficient milk production," including "no milk" or "no hope" (188). One woman reports hearing the phrase "crazy lady" (189). Another hears her pump speak the name of the comedian Tina Fey (194). Altogether, Cooper-Rompato understands the pump voices as an externalization of a mother's anxieties, which can take on a wide range of subject matter. Along these lines, one blogger understands the breast pump as "a window to her unconscious, a kind of supernatural or spiritual connection seeking to advise her" (199). In validating the perspectives of her research subjects, Cooper-Rompato depathologizes such acts of mad listening, highlighting instead the significance of the talking breast pump as an example of unruly phenomenology.
23. My own unruly bodymind becomes similarly stuck on repeated words and phrases. A few years ago, the expression "gravy train" came into my head suddenly and parked itself there. The phrase was meaningless to me, though this did not prevent me from ruminating on it. These two words fascinated me for reasons unknown. Perhaps it is the assonance of "gray" and "tray." Or perhaps there is some deeper psychological reason related to the semantic content. Though I had no emotional connection to this image, the thought was so relentlessly repetitive that I was forced to interpret it in every possible permutation. I looked for inciting events at the crossroads of food and finance. I thought about gravy and trains as separate entities. I discovered that the phrase belonged to a popular brand of dog food. I searched for evidence of childhood trauma. I wondered if maybe I felt that I was undeserving of success at the time this phrase dawned on me like I was taking the easy route,

riding the gravy train. Unlike the sounds of the talking breast pump, however, these words had no direct relevance to my life, that I could tell. They simply produced in me a kind of aesthetic frisson, of the "cellar door" variety. Like earworms, these intrusive phrases are another example of sonic stickiness, but the difference here is that instead of an external sound clinging to me, I hear these sounds intrasubjectively as internal dialogue, in my own voice. Not only are the words heard mentally, but they are also embodied as subvocalizations in the larynx, where small vocal muscles move in correspondence with internal speech. If you have ever experienced intrusive thoughts, especially those that are far less benign than this example, you will know how hard it is to accept them and not try to suppress or neutralize them. They are called trains of thought for a reason. Even while talking to someone, or trying to read, this particular phrase would chug along beneath the surface of consciousness: gravy train, gravy train, gravy train, gravy train, gravy train, gravy train. In this way, mad listening is often a multi-focal listening, being with two or more sounds at once, the ones in here and the ones out there, and everything in between. It lingers in the threshold where language passes over into sound and vice versa, at the point of semantic satiation.

24. Mad listening involves such literal acts of sonic subversion as spoonerism, wherein the first letters of adjacent words are swapped: "to tease one's ears" becomes "to ease one's tears," and "to listen here" becomes "to hiss and leer." Such wordplay does not just undermine the hegemony of normative grammar, but tears at the roots (or perhaps "rears at the toots") of linearity, rationality, and order. This time last year, for a matter of weeks, I was so immersed in the habit of spoonerizing that it became something of a mad praxis, to the extent that I could not stop mentally swapping letters around, and this caused me a great deal of anxiety. In my head, other people's words echoed in reverse-order, mostly as nonsense, with occasional blips of meaning—the title of a movie like *First Cow* becoming *Cursed Foe*, for example. Often, these semi-successful spoonerisms will send me into lateral thoughts of cursed cows and first foes, then onward to first curses and first kisses. At the expense of my ability to focus while falling down deep wells of distraction and abstraction, this habit of listening for

altered combinations of sound emerges as a potent reminder of language's power to remake worlds.

25. In his essay "Earslips: Of Mishearings and Mondegreens," literary Steven Connor echoes my earlier claim that "all hearing is mishearing" (par. 29). Tracing the etymology of the word "mishearing," he notes that early uses carried a more active connotation, implying deliberate acts of auditory disobedience, unlike the simple mondegreen or the misheard song lyric. The poets and coauthors David Huebert and Andy Verboom have characterized deliberate mishearings as "full mondegreens," which refers to their formal approach of misconstruing and reshaping canonical poems to challenge their representational politics, or as Verboom puts it, "to bite the heads off some fathers" (par. 4). They rewrite William Carlos Williams's poem "The Red Wheelbarrow," for example, with the misheard title: "The Dead Feel Narrow." On the other side, routine and systematic mishearings are fraught with epistemic violence and can be a form of silencing. Legal scholar James Parker and curator Joel Stern remind us that mishearing is also "an auditory effect of colonialism," wherein white ears disregard Indigenous testimony (19). Speaking to the ethics of the full mondegreen, Huebert acknowledges that "there are many other poets and poems whose mondegreening by me would be a violent colonizing enterprise" (par. 4). As such, he chooses his mishearings carefully, grappling with source poems whose politics warrant thorough pushback. Rather than an unwillingness to hear, then, mad listening should model a willingness to hear differently—in defiance to, and not compliance with, systems of oppression. In doing so, the mad listener might work towards rethinking, rewriting, and re-sounding mad representation. Recently, I heard Elton John's "Madman Across the Water" for the first time, and searched for the song on a misheard lyrics website. There, someone has written the following mondegreen: "get a load of him, he's sewing sand."
26. In a recent article by disability scholar Lennard J. Davis, the author suggests that Deaf culture is less concerned with unheard sounds than it is with questions of access: "availability of interpreters, less discrimination, and better ways to communicate using technology," for example (par. 3). Davis goes on to say that his Deaf parents would sometimes "recount the inevitable story about someone who got their hearing back and was driven crazy by all

the ambient noise in the world—cars, trucks, horns, rumbles, and even, yes, loud music and screeching birds" (par. 3). Here, as you might have noticed, Davis runs a red light through the intersection of deafness and madness. As disability scholar Christopher Krentz reminds us, these two categories have been conflated since ancient times: "Aristotle is credited with saying that, of all the senses, hearing contributes most to intelligence and knowledge. The Romans classified deaf people who did not speak with the insane" (41). Moreover, many deaf people were incarcerated in nineteenth-century "lunatic asylums." Mad listening must attend to this shared history of deaf madness and mad deafness.

27. In his autobiographical novel *A Journey Round My Skull*, Frigyes Karinthy provides a firsthand account of a craniotomy (or what used to be called trepanation), which he underwent after experiencing auditory hallucinations of passing trains. His description of the procedure is one of the most evocative and haunting sonic testimonies that one could imagine. Karinthy writes: "There was an infernal scream as the steel plunged into my skull. It sank more and more rapidly through the bone, and the pitch of its scream became louder and more piercing every second" (216). Then, he reports a "straining sensation, a feeling of pressure, a cracking sound, and a terrific wrench," as pieces of bone are broken off from his skull (220). "Each cracking sound," he says, "reminded me of taking the lid off a jam-jar, while the process as a whole was like splitting open a wooden packing-case, plank by plank (220). Karinthy's account provides invaluable historical context for an exceptionally brutal example of mad listening. As the early modernist Dolly Mackinnon tells us: "The historical archive remains redolent with recoverable aspects of historical soundscapes," and "the political economy of sounds, silences, and noise is an innovative way to reclaim diverse cultural voices through partial past soundscapes" (101). Accordingly, mad listening should attune to this wider project of reclamation by way of centering the testimonies of people who have survived psychiatric and medical intervention.

28. A phenomenology of mad listening risks locating madness squarely within the individual, whereas the outer world of sound can be seriously crazy-making, from the idling of diesel engines to the advertisements that play at double-volume, or the once-innocuous hum of the refrigerator, which now moans and wails like a vengeful

ghost. The list goes on: there is the evil laughter of seagulls, the nightly sirens, the neighbour's bad taste in music, the everlasting construction noise, the hundred-decibel squeal of the skytrain, not to mention the sound technologies that have been weaponized and turned on the public, like the infamous Mosquito Device, which the company describes as an "ultrasonic anti-loitering solution used to disperse unwanted homeless and youth gatherings" (n.pag). Writing about this device, sound studies scholar Mitchell Akiyama says that young people have found a way of reclaiming this sound by using it as a cellphone ringtone that most teachers are unable to hear (466). Akiyama concludes, however, that "this détournement does not amount to any real or practical immunity to sound," but instead has the unintended consequence of increasing prejudice against these antiauthoritarian youths. To listen madly is to take such risks, in full awareness that acts of resistance will always be met with resistance.

29. Mad listening and queer listening share many qualities. Transdisciplinary scholar Nick Walker coined the term "neuroqueer" to identify the point at which queerness and neurodivergence meet. To engage in neuroqueering, writes Walker, is to queer "one's own neurocognitive processes (and one's outward embodiment and expression of those processes) by intentionally altering them in ways that create significant and lasting increase in one's divergence from prevailing cultural standards of neuronormativity and heteronormativity" (n.pag). According to feminist and queer studies scholar Sara Ahmed, a queer politics of disorientation seeks to make the familiar strange, and "might even find joy and excitement in the horror" of disalignment (4). As philosopher Karoline Feyertag puts it, "at the core of the question of dizziness and queerness we find trouble in the sense of not feeling at ease with or in a given situation, feeling discomfort, disorientation and tumult—and also feeling a certain 'gender trouble,' a trouble of knowing where to belong" (par. 13). I relate this compound description to my own experience of dizziness and queerness, partly owing to an inner ear impairment that I have had since childhood, in combination with partial hearing loss, leading to bouts of mild vertigo. These auditory phenomena are analogous to my sense of genderqueerness, to my vertiginous sense of self, which often feels confusing and overwhelming, but also joyful and

exciting, in Ahmed's sense. Vertigo can be played with in the same way that gender can. I walk across the room as though strutting in stilettos for the first time, reaching out to walls and chairs to hold myself upright.

30. Another recent film, *Memoria* (2021) by Apichatpong Weerasethakul, follows a woman named Jessica Holland who hears a mysterious banging noise that cannot be heard by others, and consequently, she believes herself to be going mad. Like Kafka's mole, she tries to locate the origin of the sound to no avail, going so far as to recreate it in a recording studio, where she tells the audio engineer to imagine an enormous ball of concrete falling into a well. To my ears, it sounds like a combination of a bass drum, a door slam, and a controlled explosion. As if to taunt and trigger me, my fireplace has recently begun to make a very similar sound. In an unpredictable span of time after being shut off, the metal vent of my chimney will suddenly expand, creating a tremendous boom. After many nights beside the exploding fireplace, my startled response has not acclimatized in the slightest, even as I wait in nervous anticipation. And yet, in some sense, I am grateful for this disturbance, since it has helped me to retrain and reprocess other sounds that have startled me in the past.
31. As a veteran of panic attacks, I know when one is about to arrive by the sudden muffling of the world, like invisible hands held over my ears: a sense of fullness, an accompanying feeling of dizziness, and a familiar walls-closing-in sensation. My sight seems tilt-shifted and my hearing seems phase-shifted, and for a few minutes, everything is indistinct and unreal. Then comes the feeling that something worse is about to happen, though it never does. From the experiences I have collected in this essay, one should not get the impression, however, that mad listening is always panic-driven or pathological. Indeed, there are thousands of playlists available online devoted to calming anxiety. I prefer to listen to binaural beats in the delta range, a low tone that pulses at 2.5hz, which helps me regulate my anxiety. These tones have been called digital drugs, and some even claim that binaural beats can simulate the effects of actual psychedelics. Predictably, this trend has been subject to moral panic from parents who are wary of the potential dangers of so-called "i-dosing." As a freely available resource, binaural beats are at once a form of self-care and

a mad methodology, allowing listeners to experiment with perception and delight in disorientation, just as I have invited you to do throughout this chapter.

Notes

1. The experimental structure of this chapter is emboldened by a number of formally fragmentary works at the crossroads of autobiography and essay, including Wayne Koestenbaum's *The Queen's Throat: Opera, Homosexuality And The Mystery Of Desire* (1993), Kathleen Stewart's *Ordinary Affects* (2007), Maggie Nelson's *Bluets* (2009), Kier-La Janisse's *House of Psychotic Women: An Autobiographical Topography of Female Neurosis in Horror and Exploitation Films* (2012), Anne Carson's *The Albertine Workout* (2014), Susan Howe's *Debths* (2017), and Lewis Hyde's *A Primer for Forgetting: Getting Past the Past* (2019). I have also found inspiration in the audio essays of contemporary artists and philosophers such as Lawrence Abu Hamdan, Justin Barton, and Mark Fisher.
2. The audio version of this chapter is available here: https://www.notesonmadlistening.com/.
3. As Lisa Blackman writes in *Immaterial Bodies* (2012), the concept of synaesthesia has undergone a political reinvention, away from its pathologized origins, and toward the purpose of challenging "the hierarchization of the senses historically associated with the individualized body where the senses have been distinguished according to divisions made between the higher and lower, distant and contact, civilized and primitive, and even mind and body" (136).

Epilogue

Many of the concepts discussed in this book come together in Simon McBurney's popular play *The Encounter* (2016). The performance is based on an autobiographical account of an American photographer named Loren McIntyre who travels to the Javari Valley in Brazil in 1969 and encounters the Mayoruna tribe. As one of the better-known examples of headphone theatre, *The Encounter* is a one-man performance in which McBurney uses a dummy head to record binaural sounds on stage which are then transmitted to audience members' headsets. This recording technology has also been called a "head simulator," which by this point in my analysis should set off familiar alarm bells. As Alexis Soloski of the *Guardian* puts it: "McBurney describes how McIntyre chances upon the tribe, follows its members deep into the jungle, and receives telepathic messages from the headsman. These messages are beamed directly into his mind just as McBurney's speeches are beamed directly into ours" (n.pag). This study has attempted to isolate this *direct beam* in order to determine its function, along with its functional limitations. What telepathic messages do these productions aspire to share?

Throughout the preceding chapters, I have addressed six primary themes: mad phenomenology, simulated madness, intersubjective empathy, acoustic interiority, aural diversity, and representational conventions. Between and beyond these topics, however, is the matter of how each of these phenomena overlap. In each of my case studies, one

M. Tomkinson, *Sound and Sense in Contemporary Theatre*,
https://doi.org/10.1007/978-3-031-78034-9

insurmountable problem has been what Lisa Blackman refers to as a fascination with the "boundaries between the 'me' and the 'not-me'" and the "mimetic desire" to collapse this dividing line ("Mental Touch" 2). Recall the acousmatic wall in *The Eradication of Schizophrenia in Western Lapland*, which provides the audience with a physical analogy for voice hearing, or the headphones in *Her Long Black Hair* and *Here are the Fragments*, which work towards the same purpose. These formal devices have been shown to play different but essential roles in the aestheticization of madness—the potential harms of which I have also tried to illuminate.

Citing Pamela Thurshwell, Blackman describes the fantasy of direct mental access as an "erotics of mind-melding" (12). The term I have used for the culmination of this fantasy—in which audience members are encouraged to hold up their end of the simulatory bargain by suspending disbelief—is "factitious listening." This habit of "trying on" mad phenomenal experiences by temporarily adopting a certain subjective position has been a consistent feature in each of my chapters. In Chapter 3, this entailed bearing witness to an experimental therapeutic modality; in Chapter 4, sound artists crafted a live Foley soundscape to represent Ophelia's mad point of audition, and Cardiff's soundwalk invited audience members to listen madly alongside a walking narrator; in Chapter 5, a variety of immersive techniques served to approximate an ambient experience of voice hearing. Building resonances between mad studies, sound studies, and theatre studies, this project has advanced an array of critical concepts: mad auralities, mad listening, and the mad point of audition.

Such disciplinary crossroads, however, are not altogether new. As evidenced by the many scholarly citations and connections drawn throughout this book, my research builds from interdisciplinary scholarship and activist discourse spanning disability theory, feminist theory, critical race theory, queer theory, affect theory, and more. Adding to existing conversations around the philosophy of intersubjectivity, this study has grappled with specific problems in this domain related to dramaturgical conventions in contemporary theatre. It is no wonder that a concept such as mad aural simulation, which relies so heavily on utopian fantasies of shared perception (in the name of empathy, no less), would have received minimal critical attention up until this point. On this front, media studies scholars such as Carolyn Birdsall and Senta Siewert were the first to draw my attention to this subject area, and they remain the foremost scholars on the intersection between mad-sonic representation in the context of film and radio. It is their focus on sound technologies which lends this study its formal grounding in the sound design techniques used by each of the productions in question. The concept of mad auralities has also played a large part in determining the chosen case studies, which explicitly emphasize "hearing and listening madly" over "sounding mad" (though the latter also pertains).

Though popular mental health musicals also reflect these themes on a larger scale, the distinctive listening environments established by these high-impact but smaller-scale productions are similarly steeped in simulatory logics. As such, they furnish us with examples of the most prevalent tropes, clichés, stereotypes, and assumptions about mad auralities. This is not to say that such plays are inherently guilty of simulation, based on a predetermined assumption that all simulations are bad. More often than not, my question has been: how do they function, and what claims are being made here? It is also important to note that "simulation" is rarely a stated genre of performance or even a word that one might find on a playbill. As we have observed throughout the preceding case studies, simulatory logics have more to do with technical effects, and the ways in which we discuss these effects. More accurately, simulation could be described as an aesthetic paradigm, from which a few aspects might be borrowed, without fully subscribing to a genre. However, there are genre-like aspects to mental health plays as a whole. To the extent that they share an interest in immersing audiences in madness, the plays in question belong to a growing subgenre of dark tourism. According to Natalie Alvarez, the latter phenomenon refers to "the curious drive of tourists to visit sites of suffering, crisis, and devastation" (115). As dramatic examples of mad tourism, my case studies reflect a specific typological category that Alvarez calls "dark tourism as integration," which is "marked by a desire on the part of the tourist to integrate herself into the object of consumption and fantasy" (116).

Quoting theatre scholar Tracey Moore, Alvarez tests the limits of this approach, which imagines performance as a "veritable empathy boot camp" (163). This concept is indeed so taken for granted by practitioners of immersive dark tourism that the same familiar language appears frequently in promotional discourse. One recent example can be found in a review of the immersive asylum experience *Nellie and the Women of Blackwell* (2020), based on Nellie Bly's *Ten Days in a Mad-House* (1887), in which the author went undercover as a mental patient at the Women's Lunatic Asylum on Blackwell's Island in New York. One reviewer, Asya Gorovits, writes: "As a part of our 'mental patient bootcamp,' Nellie unscrolls a long list of reasons why someone might be admitted into a mental institution from 1864–1889; she asks us to read the ones that catch our eye [...] What started as an exciting journalistic mission soon turns dangerous and dark" (Gorovits par. 4). If one of the dangers of the empathy paradigm is that it is "predicated on the consumption of the other," as Alvarez puts it, it is precisely these acts of appropriation that I have tried to complicate in each of my chapters. In Gorovits's review, one encounters the idea of consumption in its most literal, and somewhat perturbing, form: "Nellies' crushed spirit is easy to sympathize with as we witness the abuse of patients in the asylum," writes the author (par. 4). "At various points of the journey," she adds, "I am pushed onto a scale by the nurse or left to shiver on a staircase collecting leaves and munch on a stale piece of bread" (par. 5). Though the soundscapes in my analysis have not always been so tangible as stale bread, I have tried to identify the experiential and ethical limitations of listening-as-other.

Where Gorovits notes that *Women of Blackwell* is meant "to teach us a lesson in local history and compassion," (par. 1) I am reminded of Alvarez's counterthesis, citing Peggy Phelan, that "performance might, instead, offer a way of seeing 'the positive role of unknowing in epistemic and ethical transactions'" (166). Each of my case studies has shown a similar investment in the imperative to know, and I have countered by insisting on the limitations of knowing. Thinking alongside Alvarez's research, which is grounded in scopic regimes and visibility politics, I have arrived at parallel conclusions in the realm of sound and aurality. In Chapter 2, I teased out the differences between physically knowing and conceptually understanding voice hearing through auditory representations. In Chapter 3, I parsed moments of phenomenological instability from lived sensory experiences of madness. In Chapter 4, I emphasized the importance of distinguishing material metaphors from those that lie beyond signification. In Chapter 5, I privilege enumeration over simulation as a way to represent my own experiences of mad listening, with no recourse to narrative continuity, and no imperative to recreate the auditory features of any single diagnostic condition.

Contributing to the aural diversity movement, John D'Arcy has proposed a variety of strategies for helping audiences "better understand diverse sensory experiences," as outlined in his essay, "Do You Hear What

I Hear?: Some Creative Approaches to Sharing and Simulating Diverse Hearing" (179). While I agree that such representations of sensory difference can help expose a broader spectrum of listening experiences, beyond normative assumptions, I would suggest that it is the concept of simulation that is worth troubling, if not abandoning altogether, since the very concept would seem to shore up representation from critique. Though D'Arcy recognizes a few "pitfalls of simulation," including a pervasive tendency to medicalize conditions, he alights upon one of the central contradictions of simulatory aesthetics, which are said to sometimes aim for "phenomenological realism," and at other times form "artistic impressions" (180). In short, this book has sought to demonstrate how readily the latter is mistaken for the former, and furthermore, how readily the former is mistaken for the actual.

In light of my invocation of unknowing throughout this study, perhaps it would be most appropriate to end on a note of irresolution. While writing these chapters, I have been continually nagged by a question posed by Jennifer Nash—namely: "What happens to outsider projects when they become *insider* projects?" ("Virtual Roundtable"). Since the formation of the discipline, proponents of mad studies have been cautious about the ways that the field has been integrated into academia. As a result of this process of integration, personal writing and arts-based research retain their secondary status as supplementary material to the conventional work of close analysis. Though I would have experimental arts-based research make up the entirety of this document, to pursue such methods of knowledge production and transmission fully within the book remains "an unrealistic prospect," in Alvarez's words, "since it requires an admission of inadequacy, ignorance, humility, and vulnerability—critical positions that do not lend themselves to persuasive performances of productivity, professionalism, and intellectual entrepreneurialism that seem increasingly on demand in the neoliberal university" (169). In line with the current demands of a scholarly monograph in the humanities, I have sought to reference, include, and demonstrate high degrees of sense-making and so-called rational argumentation. Yet, as my inquiries have progressed, I have realized that much of it remains, at best, an exercise in introspection. I am eager to learn more about new ways in which mad listening practices might confound our very sense of what an academic study should look and sound like.

Bibliography

Ablinger, Peter. "Palastmusik Für Infraschall Und Ultraschall." www.ablinger.mur.at/txt_palastmusik.html.

Ahmed, Sara. *Queer Phenomenology*. Duke University Press, 2006.

Akiyama, Mitchell. "Silent Alarm: The Mosquito Youth Deterrent and the Politics of Frequency." *Canadian Journal of Communication*, 35.3 (2010). https://doi.org/10.22230/cjc.2010v35n3a2261.

Alston, Adam. *Beyond Immersive Theatre*. Palgrave Macmillan, 2016.

Alston, Adam. "Melting Into Air: Dining in the Dark, Reification and the Aesthetics of Darkness." *Theatre in the Dark: Shadow, Gloom and Blackout in Contemporary Theatre* (2017): 64–87.

Altman, Robert B. *Sound Theory, Sound Practice*. Psychology Press, 1992.

Alvarez, Natalie. *Immersions in Cultural Difference: Tourism, War, Performance*. University of Michigan Press, 2018.

Amacher, Maryanne. "Psychoacoustic Phenomena in Musical Composition: Some Features of a 'Perceptual Geography.'" *Arcana III: Musicians on Music*, edited by John Zorn, 9–24. NewYork: Hips Road, 2008. http://www.sonami.net/Articles/Amacher-OAE.pdf.

Ando, Shuntaro, et al. "The Simulation of Hallucinations to Reduce the Stigma of Schizophrenia: A Systematic Review." *Schizophrenia Research*, 133.1 (2011): 8–16. https://doi.org/10.1016/j.schres.2011.09.011.

Andrews, Jonathan, et al. *The History of Bethlem*. Routledge, 2013.

Arnaud, Sabine. *On Hysteria*. University of Chicago Press, 2015.

Ballantyne, Elaine. "Doing Mad Studies: a Participatory Action Research Project to Explore the Experiences and Impacts of Being Part of a Mad People's History and Identity Course and the Relationship Between Critical Education,

M. Tomkinson, *Sound and Sense in Contemporary Theatre*,
https://doi.org/10.1007/978-3-031-78034-9

Activism and Emancipation." Diss. Queen Margaret University, Edinburgh, 2019.

Bano, Tim. "*The Eradication of Schizophrenia In Western Lapland*," *Summerhall, Edinburgh*, 27 Aug. 2018, www.summerhall.co.uk/press/the-eradication-of-schizophrenia-in-western-lapland-4/

Barnett, Laura. "The Play That Wants to Change the Way We Treat Mental Illness," *The Guardian*, 24 Mar. 2014, www.theguardian.com/lifeandstyle/2014/mar/24/play-mental-illness-eradication-schizophrenia-western-lapland-open-dialogue-hallucination.

Barrett, G. Douglas. "Window Piece: Seeing and Hearing the Music of Peter Ablinger." 2010. www.ablinger.mur.at/docs/barrett_window_piece.pdf.

Bassett, Kate. "*The Eradication of Schizophrenia in Western Lapland* at Shoreditch Town Hall, EC1," *The Times*, 17 Mar. 2014, www.thetimes.co.uk/article/the-eradication-of-schizophrenia-in-western-lapland-at-shoreditch-town-hall-ec1-cf365hc9bpc.

Baucom, Ian. "Frantz Fanon's Radio: Solidarity, Diaspora, and the Tactics of Listening." *Contemporary Literature* 42.1 (2001): 15–49.

Beckett, Samuel. *The Collected Shorter Plays of Samuel Beckett: All That Fall, Act Without Words, Krapp's Last Tape, Cascando, Eh Joe, Footfall, Rockaby and Others*. Grove/Atlantic, 2010.

Ben-moshe, Liat, Chris Chapman, and Allison C. Carey, Eds. *Disability Incarcerated: Imprisonment and Disability in the United States and Canada*. New York: Palgrave Macmillan, 2014.

Bennett, Susan. *Theory for Theatre Studies: Sound*. Bloomsbury Publishing, 2019.

Bernstein, Charles, ed. *Close Listening: Poetry and the Performed Word*. Oxford University Press, 1998.

Birdsall, Carolyn, and Senta Siewert. "Of Sound Mind: Mental Distress and Sound In Twentieth-Century Media Culture." *TMG Journal for Media History*, 16.1 (2013).

Blackman, Lisa. "Ethics, Embodiment and the Voice-hearing Experience." *Theory, Culture & Society*, 17.5 (2000): 55–74.

Blackman, Lisa. "Mental Touch." *Immaterial Bodies: Affect, Embodiment, Mediation*. Sage, 2012, pp. 54–76.

Blackman, Lisa. "Speculative Science, Threshold Experiences and Transsubjectivities." *Carpa 5 Keynote*, 13 Feb. 2018, https://nivel.teak.fi/carpa5/lisa-blackman-speculative-science-threshold-experiences-and-transsubjectivities/

Bonnet, François J. *The Order of Sounds: A Sonorous Archipelago*. MIT Press, 2019.

Braun, Johanna. *Hysterical Methodologies in the Arts*. Palgrave Macmillan, 2021.

Bregman, Albert S. *Auditory Scene Analysis: The Perceptual Organization of Sound*. Cambridge: MIT Press, 1990.

Brennan, Patrick. "*The Eradication of Schizophrenia in Western Lapland* (Shoreditch Town Hall)," *WhatsOnStage*, 14 Mar. 2014, www.whatsonstage.com/off-west-end-theatre/reviews/the-eradication-of-schizophrenia-in-western-laplan_33844.html.

Bretherick, Ruth. "The Urge to Disappear: Janet Cardiff's Audio Walks in London and New York." *Oxford Art Journal* 43.3 (2020): 427–443.

Brew-Parrish, Valeria. "Ragged Edge Online: Awareness Days" www.raggededgemagazine.com/archive/aware.htm.

Brown, Ross. *Sound Effect: The Theatre We Hear*. Bloomsbury Publishing, 2020.

Bruce, La Marr Jurelle. *How to Go Mad Without Losing Your Mind: Madness and Black Radical Creativity*. Duke UP, 2020.

Bruce, La Marr Jurelle. *How to Go Mad Without Losing Your Mind: Madness and Black Radical Creativity*. Duke University Press, 2020.

Bull, Michael, Les Back, and David Howes, eds. *The Auditory Culture Reader*. Bloomsbury Publishing, 2015.

Cardiff, Janet. *Her Long Black Hair*. Public Art Fund, 2004, https://www.publicartfund.org/exhibitions/view/her-long-black-hair/#section_3.

Carlson, Marla. "Looking, Listening, and Remembering: Ways to Walk New York after 9/11." *Theatre Journal* (2006): 395–416.

Carson, Anne. *The Albertine Workout*. New York: New Directions, 2014.

Carson, Anne. "The Gender of Sound: Description, Definition and Mistrust of the Female Voice in Western Culture." *Resources for Feminist Research*, 23.3 (1994): 24. https://www.proquest.com/docview/194882980?fromopenview=true&pq-origsite=gscholar&accountid=13800.

Cartreine, James. "Misophonia: When Sounds Really Do Make You." *Harvard Health*, 21 Apr. 2017, www.health.harvard.edu/blog/misophonia-sounds-really-make-crazy-2017042111534.

Castrodale, Mark. "Mad Studies and Mad-positive Music." *New Horizons in Adult Education and Human Resource Development* 31.1 (2019): 40–58.

Cecchetto, David, et al. *Phono-Fictions and Other Felt Thoughts: Catalyst: Eldritch Priest*. Noxious Sector Press, 2016.

Cecchetto, David. "Listening, Computation, and the Afterlife of Data." *YouTube*, uploaded by Cultural, Social and Political Thought, UVic, 28 Mar. 2020. www.youtube.com/watch?v=dfR11qvX5Ck.

Chandra, Kartik, Chuma Kabaghe, and Gregory Valiant. "Beyond Laurel/Yanny: An Autoencoder-Enabled Search for Polyperceivable Audio." *Proceedings of the 59th Annual Meeting of the Association for Computational Linguistics and the 11th International Joint Conference on Natural Language Processing (Volume 2: Short Papers)*. 2021.

Chen, Mel Y. "Brain Fog: The Race for Cripistemology." *Journal of Literary & Cultural Disability Studies* 8.2 (2014): 171–184.

Cheng, William. *Just Vibrations: The Purpose of Sounding Good*. University of Michigan Press, 2016.

Chion, Michel. "The Audiovisual Scene." *Audio-Vision: Sound on Screen*. Columbia University Press, 2019, pp. 66–97.

Chion, Michel. *The Voice in Cinema*. Columbia University Press, 1999.

Church, Kathryn. "It's Complicated': Blending Disability and Mad Studies in the Corporatising University." *Madness, Distress and the Politics of Disablement*. Policy Press, 2015. pp. 261–270.

Coleborne, Catharine. "Why Talk About Madness?" *Why Talk About Madness?* Palgrave Macmillan, Cham, 2020. pp. 1–13.

Connor, Steven. "Earslips: Of Mishearings and Mondegreens." *Listening In, Feeding Back*. Columbia University Press, 2009.

Conti, Meredith. *Playing Sick: Performances of Illness in the Age of Victorian Medicine*. Routledge, 2018.

Cooke, Anne. "The Ordinary Chaos of Psychosis." *British Journal of General Practice*, 65.637 (2015): 422. https://doi.org/10.3399/bjgp15X686245

Cooper-Rompato, Christine. "The Talking Breast Pump." *Western Folklore* (2013): 181–209.

Costa, Maddy. "*The Eradication of Schizophrenia in Western Lapland* Review: A Startling Piece of Work," *The Guardian*, 17 Mar. 2014, www.theguardian.com/stage/2014/mar/17/eradication-schizophrenia-western-lapland-review.

Coplan, Amy, and Peter Goldie, eds. *Empathy: Philosophical and Psychological Perspectives*. Oxford University Press, 2011.

Craig et al. "Avatar Therapy For Auditory Verbal Hallucinations In People With Psychosis: A Single-Blind, Randomised Controlled Trial." *The Lancet Psychiatry*, 5.1 (2018): 31–40.

Craig, Leigh Ann. "The History of Madness and Mental Illness in the Middle Ages: Directions and Questions." *History Compass*, 12.9 (2014): 729–744.

Cripps, Jody H., Ely Rosenblum, and A. Small. "Signed Music: An Emerging Inter-performative Art." *Waypoint: Proceedings of the Sixth Biennial Deaf Studies Today*, 6 (2014): 179–186.

Curtin, Adrian. *Avant-garde Theatre Sound: Staging Sonic Modernity*. Springer, 2014.

Da Costa, Beatriz, and Kavita Philip, eds. *Tactical Biopolitics: Art, Activism, and Technoscience*. MIT press, 2010.

Daly, Anya. "Intersubjectivity: Phenomenological, Psychological and Neuroscientific Intersections." *Merleau-Ponty and the Ethics of Intersubjectivity*. Palgrave Macmillan, London, 2016, pp. 173–221.

Daly, Anya. *Merleau-Ponty and the Ethics of Intersubjectivity*. London: Palgrave Macmillan, 2016.

Daniel, Drew. *The Melancholy Assemblage: Affect and Epistemology In the English Renaissance*. Fordham University Press, 2013.

D'Arcy, John. "Do You Hear What I Hear?: Some Creative Approaches to Sharing and Simulating Diverse Hearing." *Aural Diversity*. Routledge, 2022. pp. 178–186.

Davis, Lennard J. "Screening Deafness." *Los Angeles Review of Books*, www.lareviewofbooks.org/article/screening-deafness/.

Davies, William J. "Autistic Listening." *Aural Diversity*, edited by John L. Drever and Andrew Hugill, Routledge, 2022.

Derrida, Jacques, Pascale-Anne Brault, and Michael Naas. "'To Do Justice to Freud'": The History of Madness in the Age of Psychoanalysis." *Critical Inquiry*, 20.2 (1994): 227–266.

Dingwall-Jones, Christopher. "Mental Illness Between Subject and Object: Radical Empathy and Shared Subjectivity in Two Contemporary Performances." *Studies in theatre and Performance*, 38.1 (2018): 48–61.

Dorwart, Laura. "Revisiting Janet Cardiff's Central Park Audio Walk as an Ophelian Performance and Representation." *Liminalities: A Journal of Performance Studies*, 12.2 (2016): 1–15.

Douglas, Charlotte, and Paul Schmidt. *Collected Works of Velimir Khlebnikov*. Paul Scmidt (Trans.), Harvard University Press, 1987.

Drautzburg, Anja. *Towards a Poetics of the Mental Health Play*. Göttingen University Press, 2020.

Drever, John Levack. "Primacy of the Ear—But Whose Ear?: The Case for Auraldiversity in Sonic Arts Practice and Discourse." *Organised Sound*, 24.1 (2019): 85–95.

Dugalin, Istavan. "Istvan Reviews: *Here are the Fragments*." *Istvan Dugalin*, 26 Nov. 2019, https://istvandugalin.com/2019/11/25/here-are-the-fragments-theatre-centre/

Dumaresque, Renee. "Vulvodynia, it's in my Head: Mad Methods Toward Crip Coalition." *Journal of Feminist Scholarship*, 17.17 (2020): 81–105.

Dunn, Leslie C. "Ophelia's songs in Hamlet: Music, Madness, and the Feminine". *Embodied Voices: Representing Female Vocality in Western Culture*, edited by Leslie C. Dunn and Nancy A. Jones, Cambridge University Press, 1994. pp. 50–64.

ECT Collective. *Here Are The Fragments: Draft One*. 2022, https://vimeo.com/507786049.

Eghigian, Greg, ed. *The Routledge History of Madness and Mental Health*. Routledge, 2017.

Ellingson, Laura L. *Embodiment in Qualitative Research*. Routledge, 2017.

Ellis, Robert, Sarah Kendal, and Steven J. Taylor, eds. *Voices in the History of Madness: Personal and Professional Perspectives on Mental Health and Illness*. Springer Nature, 2021.

English, Lawrence. "Relational Listening: A Politics of Perception." *Contemporary Music Review*, 36.3 (2017): 127–142.

Erlmann, Veit, ed. *Hearing Cultures: Essays on Sound, Listening and Modernity*. Routledge, 2020.

Fanon, Frantz. "This is the Voice of Algeria." *A Dying Colonialism*. New York: Monthly Review, 1965, pp. 69–98.

Fanon, Frantz. *Black Skin, White Masks*. Grove Press, 2008.

Feaster, Patrick. "Phonography." *Keywords in Sound*, edited by David Novak and Matt Sakakeeny, Duke University Press, 2015, pp. 139–150.

Feyertag, Karoline. "Queering Dizziness." *On-Dizziness*, 6 Apr. 2017, www.ondizziness.com/resources-overview/queering-dizziness.

Fournier, Lauren. *Autotheory as Feminist Practice in Art, Writing, and Criticism*. MIT Press, 2021.

Fowler, Benjamin, ed. *The Theatre of Katie Mitchell*. Routledge, 2018.

Fraser, Will. "Eldritch Priest." www.thirdrailquarterly.org/eldritch-priest/.

Fretwell, Erica. *Sensory Experiments: Psychophysics, Race, and the Aesthetics of Feeling*. Duke UP, 2020.

Frieze, James. *Theatrical Performance and the Forensic Turn*. Routledge, 2019.

Gallagher, Shaun, and Dan Zahavi. *The Phenomenological Mind*. Routledge, 2020.

Gardner, Lyn. "Interactive Theatre: With Power Comes Responsibility," *The Guardian*, 12 July 2012, www.theguardian.com/stage/theatreblog/2012/jul/12/theatre1.

Gardner, Lyn. "Should Immersive Theatre Audiences Accept Greater Responsibility?," *The Guardian*, 12 Nov. 2014, www.theguardian.com/stage/theatreblog/2014/nov/12/immersive-theatre-audiences-take-responsibility-border game-the-privileged.

Gilman, Sander. *Seeing the Insane*. University of Nebraska Press, 1996.

Goodden, Sky. "Arcades as Intérieur: The Production of Distance in Sophie Calle and Janet Cardiff." Diss. OCAD University, 2010.

Goodman, Steve, Toby Heys, and Eleni Ikoniadou, eds. *Unsound: Undead*. MIT Press, 2019.

Gorovits, Asya. "Nellie and the Women of Blackwell Recreates 19th Century Horrors (Review)," *Medium*, 25 Feb. 2020, noproscenium.com/nellie-and-the-women-of-blackwell-recreates-19th-century-horrors-review-dd60425c59ea.

Hacking, Ian. "Madness: Biological or Constructed?" *The Social Construction of What*. Harvard University Press, 1999. pp. 100–124.

Hadley, Bree. *Disability, Public Space Performance and Spectatorship: Unconscious Performers*. Springer, 2014.

Halliwell, Stephen. *The Aesthetics of Mimesis*. Princeton University Press, 2009.

Harpin, Anna, and Juliet Foster, eds. *Performance, Madness and Psychiatry: Isolated Acts*. Springer, 2014.
Harpin, Anna. "'You Were an O. Your Black O in the Middle of Your Face': Madness and Catastrophe in Katie Mitchell's *Ophelias Zimmer* and *Anatomy of a Suicide*." *Contemporary Theatre Review*, 30.2 (2020): 193–210.
Harpin, Anna. *Madness, Art, and Society: Beyond Illness*. Routledge, 2018.
Hayles, N. Katherine. "Voices out of Bodies, Bodies out of Voices: Audiotape and the Production of Subjectivity." *Sound States: Innovative Poetics And Acoustical Technologies*, (1997): 74–96.
Hereditary. Directed by Ari Aster, Lionsgate, 2018.
Hill, Edwin C. *Black Soundscapes White Stages: The Meaning of Francophone Sound in the Black Atlantic*. Johns Hopkins University Press, 2013.
Home-Cook, George. *Theatre and Aural Attention: Stretching Ourselves*. Springer, 2015.
Hornstein, Gail. "Narratives of Madness, as Told From Within." *Chronicle of Higher Education*, 48.20 (2002): B7.
Howe, Susan. *Debths*. New Directions Publishing, 2017.
Huebert, David, and Andy Verboom. "Ethics in Constraint: Liberation and Determinism in the Misheard Lyric." *The Town Crier*, www.towncrier.puritan-magazine.com/full-mondegreens/.
Hugill, Andrew. *Pataphysics: A Useless Guide*. Mit Press, 2012.
Hyde, Lewis. *A Primer for Forgetting: Getting Past the Past*. Canongate Books, 2019. "Inside *The Eradication of Schizophrenia in Western Lapland*: A Short Film." *Vimeo*, uploaded by Ridiculusmus, 14 May 2014, vimeo.com/95255856.
Ingram, Richard A. "Doing Mad Studies: Making (Non)sense Together." *Intersectionalities: A Global Journal of Social Work Analysis, Research, Polity, and Practice*, 5.3 (2016): 11–17.
Irigaray, Luce. *I Love to You: Sketch of a Possible Felicity in History*. Routledge, 2016.
Janisse, Kier-La. *House Of Psychotic Women: An Autobiographical Topography of Female Neurosis in Horror and Exploitation Films*. SCB Distributors, 2015.
Johnston, Matthew. "When Madness Meets Madness: Insider Reflections on Doing Mental Health Research." *International Journal of Qualitative Methods*, 18 (2019): 1609406919835356.
Joker. Directed by Todd Phillips, Warner Bros., 2019.
Kane, Brian. *Sound Unseen: Acousmatic Sound in Theory and Practice*. Oxford University Press, 2014.
Kaplan, Ellen W. "The Cage Is My Mind: Object and Image in Depicting Mental Illness On Stage." *Studies in Theatre & Performance*, 25.2 (2005).
Karinthy, Frigyes. *A Journey Round My Skull*. New York Review of Books, 2008.

Kendrick, Lynne, and David Roesner, eds. *Theatre Noise: The Sound of Performance*. Newcastle upon Tyne: Cambridge Scholars Publishing, 2011.

Kendrick, Lynne. "Listening: Headphone Theatre and Auditory Performance." *Theatre Aurality*. Palgrave Macmillan, London, 2017, pp. 51–71.

Kendrick, Lynne. "Theatre Aurality: Beginnings." *Theatre Aurality*. Palgrave Macmillan, London, 2017, pp. 27–50.

Kheshti, Roshanak. *Modernity's Ear: Listening to Race and Gender in World Music*. Vol. 3. NYU press, 2015.

Kim, Christine Sun. "Elevator Pitch." *Christine Sun Kim*, www.christinesunkim.com/work/elevator-pitch/.

Klich, Rosemary. "Amplifying Sensory Spaces: The In-and Out-Puts of Headphone Theatre." *Contemporary Theatre Review*, 27.3 (2017): 366–378.

Klich, Rosemary Napier. "Of Unsound Mind and Body: Immersive Experience in Headphone Theater." *Emerging Affinities—Possible Futures of Performative Arts*, edited by Mateusz Borowski, Mateusz Chaberski and Malgorzata Sugiera, Bielefeld: transcript Verlag, 2019, pp. 107–126. https://doi.org/10.1515/9783839449066-007

Koestenbaum, Wayne. *The Queen's Throat: Opera, Homosexuality and the Mystery of Desire*. Poseidon Press, 1993.

Komporály, Jozefina. "Cripping Up is the Twenty-first's Century Answer to Blacking Up: Conversations With Kate O'Reilly on Theatre, Feminism and Disability." *Gender Forum*, 12 (2007).

Kuppers, Petra. *The Scar of Visibility: Medical Performances and Contemporary Art*. University of Minnesota Press, 2007.

Last Night in Soho. Directed by Edgar Wright, Universal, 2022.

Lease, Bryce. "Interview with Katie Mitchell." *Contemporary Theatre Review*, 30.2 (2020): 253–259.

Lentjes, Rebecca. "Nonconsensual Listening, Everyday Sexism, and the Mundanity of Trauma" 14 Feb. 2021, www.rebeccalentjes.com/.

Liegghio, Maria. "A Denial of Being: Psychiatrization as Epistemic Violence." *Mad Matters: A Critical Reader In Canadian Mad Studies*, edited by Brenda LeFrançois, Robert Menzies, and Geoffrey Reaume. Canadian Scholars' Press, 2013.

Lucas, Ilana. "Review: *Here Are the Fragments*." *Mooney on Theatre*, 23 Nov. 2019, www.mooneyontheatre.com/2019/11/23/review-here-are-the-fragments-ect-collective-the-theatre-centre/.

Macdonald, Michael. *Mystical Bedlam: Madness, Anxiety and Healing in Seventeenth-Century England*. Cambridge University Press, 1981.

MacKinnon, Dolly. "Hearing Madness and Sounding Cures: Recovering Historical Soundscapes of the Asylum." *Politiques de communication*, (2017): 77–106.

Maga, Carly. "*Here Are The Fragments* Is Immersive Theatre That's Worth The Trip." *The Star*, 23 Nov. 2019, www.thestar.com/entertainment/stage/2019/11/23/here-are-the-fragments-is-mmersive-theatre-thats-worth-the-trip.html.
Magelssen Scott. *Simming: Participatory Performance and the Making of Meaning*. University of Michigan Press 2014.
Malaspina, Cecile. *An Epistemology of Noise*. Bloomsbury Publishing, 2018.
"*Marat/Sade* (1967) + subtitles." *YouTube*, uploaded by Fidelis Scardanelli, 18 October 2012, www.youtube.com/watch?v=RJc4I6pivqg.
McKeown, Lisa. "Thoughtful Experiment." *Press Reader*, www.pressreader.com/canada/now-magazine/20191128/281956019639588.
McNay, Anna. "Shannon Yee: It's One Step Better Than Walking In Somebody Else's Shoes," www.studiointernational.com/index.php/shannon-yee-interview-reassembled-slightly-askew-life-threatening-brain-infacton.
McRuer, Robert. *Crip Theory: Cultural Signs Of Queerness And Disability*. NYU press, 2006.
McRuer, Robert, and Merri Lisa Johnson. "A Virtual Roundtable." *Journal of Literary & Cultural Disability Studies*, 8.2 (July 2014): 149, Gale Literature Resource Center, link.gale.com/apps/doc/A375817483/LitRC?u=anon~b5ce61f0&sid=googleScholar&xid=0bf21847.
Merleau-Ponty, Maurice. *Phenomenology of Perception*. Routledge, 2013.
Merleau-Ponty, Maurice. *The Visible and the Invisible*. Northwestern University Press, 1968.
Michael Clayton. Directed by Tony Gilroy, Warner Bros., 2008.
Midelfort, Erik. *A History of Madness in Sixteenth-Century Germany*. Stanford University Press, 1999.
Miron, Janet. "'Open to the Public': Touring Ontario Asylums in the Nineteenth Century." *Mental health and Canadian society: Historical perspectives*, (2006): 19–48.
Mitchell, David T., and Sharon L. Snyder. "Narrative Prosthesis and the Materiality of Metaphor." *Narrative Prosthesis*. University of Michigan Press, 2014.
Mitchell, Katie, and Julie Campbell. "Interview with Katie Mitchell." *Journal of Beckett Studies*, 8.1 (1998): 126–139.
Mitchell, Katie. *Ophelia's Zimmer*. *Vimeo*, uploaded by Schaubhne Berlin, 4 September 2018, vimeo.com/288228141/62b75e622c.
Mitchell, Katie. *The Director's Craft: A Handbook for the Theatre*. Routledge, 2008.
Montironi, Maria Elisa. "The Soundscape of *Ophelia's Zimmer/Ophelia's Room*." *Linguæ &-Rivista di Lingue e Culture Moderne*, 19.1 (2020): 133–154.

Mudry, Albert, and Robert K. Jackler. "Tracing the Origins of 'Cauliflower Ear' and Its Earlier Names over Two Millenia." *The Laryngoscope*, 131.4 (2021): E1315–E1321.

Murray, Heather. *Asylum Ways of Seeing: Psychiatric Patients, American Thought and Culture*. University of Pennsylvania Press, 2022.

Murphy, Tom. *The Mommo Plays: Brigit; Bailegangaire; A Thief of a Christmas*. Bloomsbury Publishing, 2014.

Nancy, Jean-Luc. *Listening*. Fordham UP, 2007.

Napolin, Julie Beth. *The Fact of Resonance: Modernist Acoustics and Narrative Form*. Fordham University Press, 2020.

Nelson, Maggie. *Bluets*. Wave Books 2009.

"Ophelia's Room" *Schaubühne Berlin*, www.schaubuehne.de/en/produktionen/ophelias-zimmer.html.

"Ophelias Zimmer" *The Key of It*, 26 May 2016, thekeyofit.wordpress.com/2016/05/26/ophelias-zimmer/.

Ovadija, Mladen. *Dramaturgy of Sound in the Avant-Garde and Postdramatic Theatre*. McGill-Queen's Press, 2013.

Peirce, Charles Sanders. "What is a Sign?" *Essential Pierce*, Vol. 2, Indiana University Press, pp. 5–10.

Peterkin, Allen. "Theatre Of Medicine/Staging Medicine." *Health-humanities.com*, 2022, http://health-humanities.com/2015/10/21/theatre-of-medicinestaging-medicine/.

Peterson, Dale, ed. *A Mad People's History of Madness*. University of Pittsburgh Press, 1982.

Phelan, Peggy. "Reconsidering Identity Politics, Essentialism, and Dismodernism: An Afterword." *Bodies in Commotion: Disability and Performance*, edited by Carrie Sandahl and Philip Auslander, University of Michigan Press, 2005, pp. 319–326.

Pickens, Therí Alyce. *Black Madness: Mad Blackness*. Duke University Press, 2019.

Pinch, Trevor, and Karin Bijsterveld, eds. *The Oxford Handbook of Sound Studies*. Oxford University Press, 2012.

Pine, B. Joseph, Joseph Pine, and James H. Gilmore. *The Experience Economy: Work is Theatre and Every Business a Stage*. Harvard Business Press, 1999.

Poe, Edgar Allan. *Complete Stories and Poems of Edgar Allan Poe*. Doubleday, 2012.

Porter, Roy. *A Social History of Madness: The World through the Eyes of the Insane*. E.P. Dutton, 1989.

Pressnitzer, Daniel, et al. "Auditory Perception: Laurel and Yanny Together At Last." *Current Biology*, 28.13 (2018): R739–R741.

Ratner, Megan. "Janet Cardiff," 11 November 2004, https://www.frieze.com/article/janet-cardiff.

Read, John, Loren R. Mosher, and Richard P. Bentall, eds. *Models of Madness: Psychological, Social and Biological Approaches to Schizophrenia*. Psychology Press, 2004.

Reaume, Geoffrey. "How is Mad Studies Different from Anti-psychiatry and Critical Psychiatry?" *The Routledge International Handbook of Mad Studies*. Routledge, 2021, pp. 98–107.

Reaume, Geoffrey. "Mad People's History." *Radical History Review* 2006.94 (2006): 170–182.

Raudive, Konstantins. *Breakthrough: An Amazing Experiment in Electronic Communication With the Dead*. Smythe, 1971.

Read, Tim. "The Eradication of Schizophrenia in Western Lapland" *Civilian Theatre*, 18 Feb. 2015, civiliantheatre.com/2015–2/the-eradication-of-schizophrenia-in-western-lapland/.

Reid, Jenna, et al. "Mobilizing Mad Art in the Neoliberal University." *Journal of Literary & Cultural Disability Studies*, 13.3 (2019): 255–272.

Redikopp, Sarah. "Out of Place, Out of Mind: Min(d)ing Race in Mad Studies Through a Metaphor of Spatiality." *Canadian Journal of Disability Studies*, 10.3 (2021): 96–118.

"Residency Page: The Theatre Centre." *Theatrecentre.org*, 2022, https://theatrecentre.org/residency/residency-page-template/.

"Responses to *The Eradication of Schizophrenia in Western Lapland*." *Vimeo*, uploaded by Ridiculusmus, 14 May 2014, https://vimeo.com/75918173

"Ridiculusmus Virtual Trilogy Dialogue As The Embodiment of Love" New Adelphi Theatre, www.newadelphitheatre.co.uk/event/ridiculusmus-virtual-trilogy-dialogue-as-the-embodiment-of-love/.

Robinson, Dylan. *Hungry Listening: Resonant Theory for Indigenous Sound Studies*. U of Minnesota Press, 2020.

Rost, Katharina. 2011. "Intrusive Noises: The Performative Power of Theatre Sounds." *Theatre Noise: The Sound of Performance*, edited by Lynne Kendrick and David Roesner, Newcastle upon Tyne: Cambridge Scholars Publishing, 2011, pp. 44–45.

Russo, Jasna, and Peter Beresford. "Between Exclusion and Colonisation: Seeking a Place for Mad People's Knowledge in Academia." *Disability & Society*, 30.1 (2015): 153–157.

Sacks, Oliver. *The Man Who Mistook His Wife for a Hat and Other Clinical Tales*. Knopf, 2021.

Samuels, Ellen. *Fantasies of Identification: Disability, Gender, Race*. NYU Press, 2014.

Schafer, Raymond Murray. *The Soundscape: Our Sonic Environment and the Tuning of the World*. Rochester, VT: Destiny Books, 1994.

Schaub, Mirjam. "The Affective Experience of Space." *The Oxford Handbook of Sound and Image in Western Art* (2016): 214.

Schaub, Mirjam. *Janet Cardiff: The Walk Book*. Walther Koenig, 2005.

Schaubühne Berlin. "*Ophelias Zimmer*: Proben-Trailer der Schaubühne Berlin," 1 Dec. 2015, https://www.youtube.com/watch?v=H-9CGCtyOu4.

Schreber, Daniel Paul. *Memoirs Of My Nervous Illness*. New York Review of Books, 2000.

Schrimshaw, Will. *Immanence and Immersion: On the Acoustic Condition in Contemporary Art*, Bloomsbury Academic & Professional, 2017. ProQuest Ebook Central, https://ebookcentral-proquest-com.proxy.lib.sfu.ca/lib/sfu-ebooks/detail.action?docID=5014620.

Schrimshaw, Will. *Immanence and Immersion: On the Acoustic Condition in Contemporary Art*. Bloomsbury, 2017.

Schulze, Daniel. *Authenticity in Contemporary Theatre and Performance: Make it Real*. Bloomsbury Publishing, 2017.

Sconce, Jeffrey. *Haunted Media: Electronic Presence from Telegraphy To Television*. Duke University Press, 2000.

Seikkula, Jaakko. "Inner And Outer Voices In The Present Moment Of Family And Network Therapy." *Journal of Family Therapy*, 30.4 (2008): 478–491.

Shaughnessy, Nicola. "The Arts and Developmental Psychopathology." *The Wiley Handbook of Developmental Psychopathology* (2017): 61.

Showalter, Elaine. *Representing Ophelia: Women, Madness, and the Responsibilities of Feminist Criticism*. Macmillan, 1994.

Showalter Elaine. *The Female Malady: Women Madness and English Culture 1830–1980*. Virago 1987.

Siisiäinen, Lauri. *Foucault and the Politics of Hearing*. Routledge, 2012.

Silver Linings Playbook. Directed by David Russell, Alliance Films, 2013.

Silverman, Arielle. "Disability Simulations: What Does the Research Say?" *Nfb.org*, 1 June 2017, nfb.org//sites/default/files/images/nfb/publications/bm/bm17/bm1706/bm170602

Soloski, Alexis. "*The Encounter* Review: Simon McBurney's Revolution in the Head." *The Guardian*, 30 Sept. 2016, www.theguardian.com/stage/2016/sep/29/the-encounter-review-simon-mcburney-revolution-headphones.

Spandler, Helen, and Jill Anderson, eds. *Madness, Distress and the Politics of Disablement*. Policy Press, 2015.

Spandler, Helen, and Dina Poursanidou. "Who is Included in the Mad Studies Project?" *The Journal of Ethics in Mental Health*, 10 (2019).

Spencer, Amy. "Literary Thresholds: Exploring the Edges of Ambient Literature." *Matlit: Materialidades Da Literatura*, 6.1 (2018): 149–158.

Split. Directed by M. Night Shyamalan, Universal, 2017.

Steingo, Gavin, and Jim Sykes, eds. *Remapping Sound Studies*. Duke University Press, 2019.

Sterne, Jonathan. "Hearing." *Keywords in Sound*, edited by David Novak and Matt Sakakeeny, Duke University Press, 2015, pp. 65–77.

Sterne, Jonathan. *The Sound Studies Reader*. Routledge, 2012.

Stewart, Kathleen. *Ordinary Affects*. Duke University Press, 2007.

Stoever, Jennifer Lynn. *The Sonic Color Line: Race and the Cultural Politics of Listening*. Vol. 17. New York University Press, 2016.

Talbot, R. J. "Reflections On *The Eradication Of Schizophrenia In Western Lapland*: A Conversation Between David Woods and Jon Haynes of Ridiculusmus with Commentary by Richard Talbot." *Performing Psychologies : Imagination, Creativity and Dramas of the Mind*, edited by Nicola Shaughnessy and Philip Barnard, Bloomsbury, 2019, pp. 167–187.

The Soloist. Directed by Joe Wright, DreamWorks, 2009.

Thomaidis, Konstantinos. *Theatre and Voice*. Macmillan International Higher Education, 2017.

Thomas, Philip and Eleanor Longden. "Phenomenology in a Different Key: Narrative, Meaning, and Madness." *Philosophy, Psychiatry, & Psychology*, 22.3 (2015): 187–192. *Project MUSE*, https://doi.org/10.1353/ppp.2015.0031.

Thompson, Marie, and Ian Biddle, eds. *Sound, Music, Affect: Theorizing Sonic Experience*. A&C Black, 2013.

Thorpe, Suzanne. "Composing With Resonance, Sounding the Inaudible, and Listening for More-Than-One." *Distributed Perception: Resonances and Axiologies*, edited by Natasha Lushetich and Iain Campbell. Routledge, 2021, pp. 82–98.

Titchkosky, Tanya, Devon Healey, and Rod Michalko. "Blindness Simulation and the Culture of Sight." Journal of Literary & Cultural Disability Studies, 13.2 (2019): 123–139, https://muse.jhu.edu/article/725084

Venn, Jon. "Hearing Voices, Seeing Visions: Hallucination, Space and Mad Experience." *Madness in Contemporary British Theatre*. Palgrave Macmillan, 2021, pp. 67–113.

Venn, Jon. *Madness in Contemporary British Theatre: Resistances and Representations*. Springer Nature, 2021.

Verma, Neil. *Theater of the Mind: Imagination, Aesthetics, and American Radio Drama*. University of Chicago Press, 2019.

Wald, Christina. *Hysteria, Trauma and Melancholia: Performative Maladies In Contemporary Anglophone Drama*. Springer, 2007.

Walker, Nick. "Neuroqueer: An Introduction." *Neuroqueer*, https://neuroqueer.com/neuroqueer-an-introduction/.

Weber, Bruce. "An Endlessly Repeated Tale That Never Reaches an Ending." *The New York Times*, www.nytimes.com/2002/10/15/theater/theater-review-an-endlessly-repeated-tale-that-never-reaches-an-ending.html.

Westall, Mark. "FUTURO-A: The World's Highest Experiment in Empathy Engineering on Flight LH448" *FAD Magazine*, 4 Feb. 2019, http://fadmagazine.com/2019/02/04/futuro-a-the-worlds-highest-experiment-in-empathy-engineering-on-flight-lh448/.

White, Gareth. "On Immersive Theatre." *Theatre Research International*, 37.3 (2012): 221–235.

Woods, David, and Jon Haynes. *The Eradication of Schizophrenia in Western Lapland*. Bloomsbury Publishing, 2014.

Woods, David. "Breakthrough moments: Open Dialogue in the Ridiculusmus play *The Eradication of Schizophrenia in Western Lapland*." *Context: The Magazine for Family Therapy and Systemic Practice*, 138 (2015): 36–38.

"Yes, Yes, Yes" *Ridiculusmus*, 1 Apr. 2013, www.ridiculusmus.com/shows/past-shows/yes-yes-yes/.

Zeavin, Hannah. *The Distance Cure: A History of Teletherapy*. MIT Press, 2021.

Zizek, Slavoj. *Living in the End Times*. Verso Books, 2011.

Index

M. Tomkinson, *Sound and Sense in Contemporary Theatre*,
https://doi.org/10.1007/978-3-031-78034-9

The manufacturer's authorised representative in the EU is Springer Nature Customer Service Centre GmbH, Europaplatz 3, 69115 Heidelberg, Germany. If you have any concerns regarding our products, please contact ProductSafety@springernature.com

Printed and bound by CPI Group (UK) Ltd, Croydon, CR0 4YY
01/10/2026
02225978-0014